THE MOTEN METHOD

FOR

Knee Pain Relief

The Moten Method for Knee Pain Relief

Why Standard Care Fails and What Actually Heals

Renee Moten

Published by Game Changer Publishing

Paperback ISBN: 979-8-90158-099-8

Hardcover ISBN: 979-8-90158-103-2

Digital ISBN: 979-8-90158-104-9

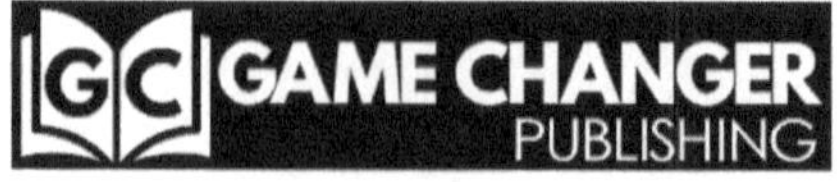

*This book is dedicated to my clients, the true architects of the Moten Method.
You trusted me with your pain, your frustration, and your hope at a time
when answers were limited and options felt bleak. You showed me what
actually works, not in theory, but in real life.
And especially to Aretha,
who tuned into my online exercise class in 2019 and stayed when no one else
did. For an entire year, she was the only one who showed up. Her consistency
helped me stay the course when quitting would have been easier. Eight years
later, she is still with me.
This book exists because of all of you.
Your Knee Keeper For Life*

Renee Moten

ADVANCE PRAISE

wrong. I had never been taught to address and reduce inflammation first before doing anything else. That realization was pivotal.

I learned that I could change my thinking and take control of my healing rather than depending on doctors, physical therapists, and insurance companies to dictate my care.

—Gayle M.

I had suffered from right knee pain for many years. My morning ritual was to make coffee and take Tylenol every day. After six months, Tylenol was no longer part of my daily routine.

That change was due to the Moten Method.

—Margery Byfield

After going to specialists for crippling knee pain and experiencing no relief from pain medication, cortisone shots, or physical therapy, I found Renee and the Moten Method. It changed my life. In just a few months, I was able to climb stairs, go for walks, and enjoy family vacations again.

I have been knee pain free for over four years.

—Jennifer Goodman

Before reading The Moten Method for Knee Pain Relief, my knee pain was so intense that I had trouble walking and it was affecting my sleep. I had tried everything, including physical therapy and strengthening exercise videos, but nothing helped because I was not addressing the real issue.

This book lays out a six-step system that no one had ever explained to me before. It is a clear, easy-to-apply approach to knee pain reduction that showed me why nothing I tried before was working and how to finally get out of pain.

When I reached Step 2 of the Moten Method, which focuses on the lymphatic system, I noticed a reduction in pain almost immediately. As I progressed through the stages outlined in the book, my knees continued to improve. Today, I am back to jogging and hiking pain free.

This book gave me clarity and real relief when I felt like I was running out of options.

—Naheed Oberfeld

For the first time, I understood why my struggles with right knee pain were happening after reading The Moten Method for Knee Pain by Renee Moten. Her first chapter, in which she shares her own pain and struggles, deeply resonated with me.

Chapter 5 was a miraculous read and gave me practical steps and tools to help alleviate pain, including exfoliation, hydrotherapy, and lymph drainage. The chapters on stabilizing and strengthening the body also helped me return to an active lifestyle.

The entire book is full of information to restore the body and live life fully active and pain free without surgery. Worth the read.

—L. C.

I have suffered from a meniscus tear in my knee for many years. After using Renee Moten's knee pain recipe for exfoliation and lymph-draining massage, I experienced a dramatic improvement in my mobility, including going up and down stairs and engaging in other exercise activities.

—Ellen Woodson

I had been struggling with a swollen, painful knee for a couple of years, and medical professionals were of no help. Fortunately, I came across the Heal My Knees website, the best thing that could have happened.

Within weeks of joining Renee's program, the swelling and knee pain disappeared. Now, more than four years later, I continue to follow Renee's recommendations for exfoliation, hydrotherapy, and lymph drainage, and as a result, my knees remain pain free.

—Nerys

NOTE FROM THE KNEE KEEPER:

Just to say thanks for buying and reading my book,
As a bonus for buying my book

Scan the QR Code to get my eBook:
"Unlocking the Secrets to Knee Pain"
and use promo code MYKNEE:

THE MOTEN METHOD

FOR

Knee Pain Relief

*Why Standard Care Fails and
What Actually Heals*

RENEE MOTEN

FOREWORD

There are moments when a book lands in your hands not by accident, but by alignment. This is one of those books.

When Renee first shared her vision for The Moten Method For Knee Pain, I knew immediately this wasn't just about knee pain. It was about reclaiming trust in the body. It was about hope. It was about empowering people to listen more deeply to their pain, their intuition, and their innate capacity to heal. It was THE method for healing.

As a transformational mentor and thought leader, I've spent years working with individuals who feel betrayed by their bodies. Pain has a way of shrinking lives. It limits movement, yes, but more than that, it limits possibility. It whispers lies: *"You're broken. This is just how it is now. Surgery is inevitable."*

Renee gently, confidently, and expertly challenges those narratives.

What makes this book so powerful is that it doesn't approach healing as a quick fix or a one-size-fits-all protocol. Instead, it honors the intelligence of the body and the wisdom that emerges when we address pain from the inside out: physically, emotionally, and energetically.

Renee bridges science, practical guidance, and deep compassion in a way that makes readers feel seen, safe, and capable.

This is not a book written from theory alone. It is written from lived experience, professional mastery, and an unwavering belief that the body is not the enemy; it is the messenger.

Within these pages, you'll find more than strategies to reduce knee pain and restore mobility. You'll find permission to slow down, to question fear-based medical narratives, and to become an active participant in your own healing journey. You'll learn how to work *with* your body instead of against it, and in doing so, you may discover strength, resilience, and freedom you didn't realize were still available to you.

If you are reading this because you're in pain, I want you to know this: you are not weak, you are not failing, and you are not out of options. Healing is not always linear, but it is always possible when approached with curiosity, patience, and the right guidance.

Renee is that guide.

I am deeply honored to support her and to introduce you to this work. May this book be a turning point not just for your knees, but for the relationship you have with your body as a whole.

With belief in your healing,

—Dana Grant, Global Transformation Mentor & Speaker

A NOTE TO THE READER

I've always believed that movement is freedom. Long before I became a personal trainer, a massage therapist, and the woman helping thousands of other women reclaim their knees, I was simply a kid who loved to run track, play softball, jump rope, and climb every tree I wasn't supposed to. That love of movement followed me into adulthood, onto soccer fields and into gyms, and eventually into the lives of people desperate to get their own movement back.

But I never imagined the thing I loved most, "movement," would be the very thing I would lose.

My journey into knee pain didn't begin with some dramatic sports injury or a collision while I was scoring the winning goal. I wish! No, it wasn't that dramatic. What should have been an ordinary moment quietly detonated into twenty years of limping, swelling, stiffness, and a revolving door of four orthopedic surgeons offering outdated methods.

For two decades, my ankles, feet, hips, and knees ran the show, and I wasn't the boss. I went from athletic and active to waking up feeling like a mummy rising from its tomb, like I was seventy when I was barely forty. Pain didn't knock; it just moved in, rearranged my furniture, and made itself comfortable.

My turning point came when I realized that the traditional orthopedic model had nothing new to say. It was the same tired playlist on repeat: Strengthen it. Brace it. Ice it. Medicate it. Inject it. And when all else fails, cut it.

That was the script, over and over. And none of it worked, not for me and not for the thousands of people I would eventually serve. Something inside me refused to believe that drugs and surgery were the only way to a pain-free life.

So, I went searching.

I attended over one hundred health and wellness classes, chasing answers like my life depended on it because, honestly, it did. Then, in 2010, everything shifted. I discovered that the source of my twenty years of knee pain… wasn't the root cause of the pain.

My real issues were hiding in plain sight: a misaligned kinetic chain starting at my ankles and a lymphatic system that had basically gone on strike. I almost fell out of my chair when the instructor said that most knee problems start at the ankle. I finally found the reason for my pain.

So, I went to work correcting these overlooked root causes. The pain that used to yell at me every morning faded into a whisper and eventually disappeared completely. My morning stiffness was gone. Pain while climbing the stairs was gone. Pain from exercise, walking, and jumping was gone. Not for a weekend. Not for a month. **Permanently.**

That is why I wrote this book.

Far too many people are told there's nothing they can do.

Far too many are handed the same tired list: physical therapy, drugs, shots, or surgery.

Far too many walk around feeling hopeless, frustrated, or dismissed when, in reality, their bodies simply need a different approach.

This book is for you if you refuse to accept stiffness, swelling, or the assumption that surgery is your destiny. If you've been told your pain is just due to "age," "weight," "arthritis," or even "bone on bone," yet deep down inside, you keep saying there *has* to be another answer, keep reading. Your instincts are correct; there is another way.

Why should you listen to me?

Because I've lived every part of this journey, I know exactly what you're facing. I've been through it myself: The limping and swollen joints. Trying to climb the stairs and having to stop. Quitting exercise programs because my knees swelled like balloons. Staggering home because I pushed myself too far on a walk.

Do any of my experiences sound like yours?

In this book, you'll learn why your pain hasn't improved, what the orthopedic world keeps overlooking, and how a few simple, strategic steps can help restore the mobility you thought was gone forever. You'll discover how to reduce inflammation naturally, realign your kinetic chain, address silent root causes, and, most importantly, how the "Moten Method" will become the gold standard for knee pain reduction.

Most of all, you'll regain something priceless: **hope**.

My journey led me to a holistic breakthrough and a patented invention that is changing how we approach knee, hip, and back pain. This book is the blueprint, a system that has been hiding in plain sight, one that millions desperately need.

So, turn the page.

Your hope and your healing begin now.

CONTENTS

1

THE ANKLE THAT TRIGGERED TWENTY YEARS OF KNEE PAIN

Every athlete knows injuries come with the territory. Some are annoying. Some are humbling. And some appear out of nowhere and try to snatch your whole future. My ankle injury wasn't glamorous or dramatic. One Saturday morning, during an over-thirty women's soccer game, I took a quick, wrong turn, and boom, my life was rerouted for the next twenty years.

I've always been a sports fanatic, and when I had my daughter, she too fell in love with sports. For a moment, it felt like the universe had finally heard my wishes.

I wanted her to experience the sports world with me, so I registered us for obstacle courses, ziplining, and joined a women's soccer team along the way. I envisioned us celebrating wins, bonding, and discussing soccer strategies. As I look back, I can see that the universe had other plans for me.

This was around 1986 or 1987, but trust me, the memory is still crisp. I was sprinting up the field, my heart racing, ready to score… Then my foot sank into a ditch I didn't see. My right ankle rolled so hard it felt like fireworks were shooting up my leg. Of course, being an athlete, I tried to stand and keep playing. My right ankle had other plans. I limped to the sideline, hoping for a quick sub, but my coach took one look at my face and gave me the look that said, "Yep… season over." *Ouch*. Physically defeated and emotionally destroyed, I drove home.

The doctor brushed it off as "just a bad sprain." But that so-called sprain damaged the ligaments in my right ankle and quietly set the stage for twenty years of knee pain.

My ankle healed "well enough," so I went back to my eleven-hour workdays, still trying to return to soccer. But my unhealed ankle kept rolling outward, causing me to almost fall. That did not stop me from returning to the field to play soccer. As athletes, we find a way to play through the discomfort. That's also probably when my "superwoman persona" was born… and trust me, she was not helpful.

Soon, the soles of my feet started hurting at work. I just shrugged it off. It only got worse. Then came the morning in 1990 when I stepped out of bed and collapsed. I couldn't stand up. At all. I had to crawl across the floor to call a foot doctor on the landline. (Remember those? No cell phones in those days.)

The diagnosis: plantar fasciitis. The treatment suggestions: surgery… shot… orthotics. I refused everything except the orthotics. The doctor also mentioned casually that my ankle "looked off." Neither of us realized that this was the first clue to the real problem

Still, I kept going. Limping. Working. Exercising. Pretending I was fine. Sound familiar?

Then came the day my right knee buckled during a squat routine, sending me straight to the floor. (I seem to be on the floor a lot.) A burning sensation shot through my knee, and all I could think was, *"What the hell just happened"*? The next day, the pain settled down, so I went on with life, completely unaware that I had just been invited into a world I'd never asked to join, a world called chronic knee pain.

Knee Note: *Your knee never randomly starts hurting for no reason.*

In 1992, I met my personal trainer. Before he would work with me, he insisted that I go to the doctor and get a diagnosis for my knee pain.

At the appointment, doctor number one bent my knee. It sounded just like Rice Krispies cereal.

He diagnosed me with patellofemoral syndrome and told me to strengthen my quads and lose weight. So, I worked the strengthening program with my personal trainer: squats, lunges, leg extensions, and duck walks with weights. My right knee hurt sometimes, but I pushed through the pain. I trained like this for five years.

Then I noticed a new, persistent pain, but it wasn't in my right knee. My left knee had started aching and swelling, and I knew my life would never be the same.

Knee Note: Performing the wrong exercises can accelerate cartilage breakdown in the knee rather than protect it. I did what the doctor told me to do. So why do I have pain in my left knee?

There were days when my knee would lock up on the stationary bike. I tried the treadmill, and my knee gave out. I went to the gym wearing two knee braces; I probably looked like some kind of bionic woman. People stared. I didn't care. I was desperate.

But nothing worked.

By 1998, I had been in pain for over 10 years. I had fulfilled my dream of becoming a personal trainer, mainly because I was trying to figure out why these exercises had started to hurt my left knee and why my right was still hurting. This year marked the opening of Functional Fitness, my personal training company.

I picked up a few clients and began working with them at the gym. The constant kneeling and getting up off the floor took a toll on both knees. To keep the swelling down, I wore ice packs under my pants every day. I iced constantly. I was limping, surviving, and pretending.

I was living a double life:

- Trainer by profession
- Patient by reality

Then came one cold, rainy morning in March 2000.

If you have knee pain, you know that rain is not your friend.

At 6:15 a.m., as I was traveling to my client's house in Washington, DC, I felt my knees stiffening up in my car. When I arrived, I got out of my car with 20 pounds of gear and stared at the nine steps between me and my client's door. Every step I took sounded like I was crunching gravel in my knee. By the time I reached the door, my knees had already started to swell. (Stairs are not our friend, either.)

My client worked out in the basement.

I told her, "You go first," because God forbid she saw me struggle to get down the stairs. As she went down ahead of me, I stepped to the top of the staircase. I grabbed both banisters so I would not fall. My knee buckled on the first step, and the shooting pain I experienced in both knees was awful.

I felt like an imposter, teaching strength while I couldn't walk downstairs without praying for divine intervention. I made it to the bottom, but I knew something had to change. Depression set in. The stress of the pain, my job, and supporting my family pushed me so far that in 2001, I ended up in the hospital.

The doctor said I was in a "thyroid storm," a potentially life-threatening reaction triggered by extreme stress. I had developed hyperthyroidism because the pain and pressure had chewed through my reserves.

My endocrinologist said I'd be on medication for life. I said, "Not on my watch."

Within a year, I was off the medication… but still battling knee pain.

In 2002, one of my clients suggested I get a pedicure. I didn't even know what a pedicure was at the time, but I went anyway. I mentioned to the therapist that I had pain in both knees. She was not familiar with working on knees, but she said she would see what she could do. The therapist finished the pedicure, slipped booties onto my feet, and then headed north, straight for my knees. The moment she started massaging them, every nerve in my body protested. I stayed through the pain, making a choice to be brave, knowing full well that walking the next day was going to be a problem.

Then came a "eureka" moment! The next morning, I stood from my bed, and the pain was gone. I had been in pain for ten years at this point, but in one day, it had disappeared.

I danced. I cried. I called the therapist and asked, "What did you do?" She told me she had performed a lymphatic drainage massage. I had never heard of that type of massage in my life.

I went back to her a few times, but the pain kept returning. The experience created a fire in me that still burns to this day: the desire to heal my body without drugs, shots, or surgery.

I reasoned that if she could get me out of pain that easily, then maybe *I* could, too.

This was the day everything changed.

It was the moment I stepped fully into being a holistic practitioner. I had received no drugs. No shots. No surgery for my knees. Just a few physical therapy sessions and a deep knowing in my spirit that Western medicine was not going to get me out of pain.

I had already seen what the Western medical system had done to my mother and my sister, how it had dismissed their pain, masked their symptoms, and offered quick fixes that never healed. I refused to follow the same road. Instead, I chose a different path, one that honored my body, intuition, and healing.

I went on a quest, seeking out massage therapists, chiropractors, acupuncturists, supplements, and diets. You name it, I tried it.

In 2005, I saw an ad from Dr. Berg. It said that, many times, pain is caused by fatigued adrenal glands. I had never heard of an adrenal gland. I learned that Dr. Berg was a chiropractic researcher who had been studying why chiropractic adjustments did not hold. In his findings, he said that what is going on inside the body dictates what happens on the outside. My knees were swollen and achy most of the time. Ice, ointments, and massage helped only a little. What I needed to focus on was how to rest my adrenals so they would stop creating more inflammation in my body.

Knee pain triggers stress. Stress triggers an inflammation response.

> **Knee Note:** *Adrenal glands, located atop the kidneys, are central to the body's stress response, releasing hormones like adrenaline (epinephrine) and cortisol to trigger the "fight-or-flight" reaction by increasing heart rate, blood sugar, and energy for immediate action, but chronic stress can overwhelm them, leading to prolonged hormone release that impacts metabolism, immunity, and mental health*

Around the same time, I met Dr. Berg, orthopedic doctor number three, took more X-rays, and told me I had "osteoarthritis in both knees and in both hips." Damn, would I ever get better? He suggested Celebrex, which I refused.

For ten more years, I kept searching.

And in 2014… I found it.

The root causes.

The missing links.

The overlooked pathways that no orthopedic specialist was ever taught to mention.

This book is not about blaming doctors or the medical system. It's about understanding the limitations of a system that was designed for acute injury and structural damage, not long-term functional pain.

2014 was the year I became knee-pain free. In 2015, I walked a 40-mile, two-day breast cancer walk without pain. I did it again in 2016.

A blister tried to ruin the moment, but listen, I was thrilled. I had solved my knee pain without drugs, shots, or surgery.

I shared my method in 2018. The first woman who tried my method emailed me the next day and said, *"Renee... my pain is gone. This can't be right."*

But it was.

And still is

And it begins with your story.

Your healing.

Your hope.

Let's begin.

2

WHY KNEE PAIN PERSISTS DESPITE TREATMENT

Many people continue to live with chronic knee pain, not because they did anything wrong but because traditional medical training has historically focused on immediate diagnosis and medication to manage symptoms. There is often less emphasis on teaching patients how to restore movement or daily function. In the U.S., medical students often receive as few as **eleven hours of formal pain education** across their entire training.[1]

Orthopedic professionals are exceptionally trained to identify and repair structural damage.[2] However, they aren't always trained to look at the **underlying movement patterns or physical habits** that keep knee pain coming back.

There is a growing gap between what standard orthopedic care offers and what people actually need to avoid the cycle of surgeries, drugs, and injections. Many are searching for a path that doesn't involve the constant fear of losing their independence or quality of life.

---

1. Malik, Zayir, James Ahn, Kathryn Thompson, and Alejandro Palma. "A Systematic Review of Pain Management Education in Graduate Medical Education." *Journal of Graduate Medical Education* 14, no. 2 (2022): 178–190. https://doi.org/10.4300/JGME-D-21-00672.1.
2. Malik et al., 2022

I created The Knee Pain Recipe to bridge this gap, moving from temporary pain relief to long-term knee resilience.

My six-step system targets the true root causes of knee pain, helping you reclaim your mobility and lifestyle without relying on prescriptions or invasive procedures. Whether you've been diagnosed with a meniscus tear or told you're bone-on-bone, relief is possible. The most effective answers often lie beyond the traditional model of care.

I see the impact of this growing gap every day, through the eyes of my clients and in the messages I receive from people around the world who are desperate for relief.

"Her daughter, feeling desperate, sent me a message through my social media page. She wrote, 'I'm looking for help with my mother. She has bone-on-bone arthritis and is always in pain, limping, and not wanting to go anywhere. She works as a warehouse checker, standing for eight hours a day. She receives doctor-prescribed injections, wears a brace, and uses topical creams.

However, as you mentioned in your video, these solutions are only temporary. I just want her to feel good again and enjoy life without constant pain.'"

This wasn't just another message in my social media inbox; it reflected the experiences of countless others. People are searching for hope and praying for solutions. They turn to my pages for answers for themselves and their loved ones. Knee pain doesn't just impact the individual; it affects the whole family. No one wants to witness the suffering of someone they love, least of all their mother.

Mothers chasing children, athletes chasing goals, women enduring chronic knee pain, men determined to stay active, and anyone trapped in a system that has quietly let them down all deserve a clear path forward, not a lifetime subscription to pain. So why are we expected to endure discomfort for five, ten, or even twenty years?

That question sent me investigating what actually drives this industry. What, exactly, have they learned that keeps our family members in pain?

The condition known as osteoarthritis was officially named in 1890 by Sir Archibald Edward Garrod. Yes, 1890. That means over 135 years have passed from horse-drawn carriages to smartphones, from rotary phones to artificial intelligence, and yet, from 1890 to 2026, there is still *no cure* for osteoarthritis. Let that sink in. We can FaceTime across the globe, but we can't figure out how to reduce knee pain without the drugs, shots, and surgery.

Why is that?

What I later discovered was devastating. After an osteoarthritis diagnosis, many doctors believe there is nothing to do except *manage* the problem with medications, injections, physical therapy, and eventually surgery. Translation: "Welcome to the system."

I was stunned. Because the moment osteoarthritis enters the conversation, the focus seems to shift from solving the problem to managing your expectations. Pain becomes something you're taught to tolerate, monitor, and politely live with, rather than question, challenge, or resolve.

And that… never sat right with me.

> **Knee Note:** *All chronic knee and hip pain over three years will eventually turn into Osteoarthritis because of the chronic inflammation*

Now, where did the idea originate that strengthening leg muscles could alleviate knee problems and pain? This notion gained traction in the 1980s and 1990s.

What doctors had begun to notice is that when someone experiences knee problems, their quadriceps are usually weak. This is not rocket science. If my knees hurt, I won't exercise, which means my quadriceps will be weak. Unfortunately, they concluded that you need to strengthen your quadriceps to protect the joint.

Since the 1980s, this has been the standard approach to helping people manage pain. I remember back in the 1990s, when I had knee pain, I was given the same advice: strengthen your leg muscles and lose weight. This is the same advice being given to people today in 2026. It didn't help me back in 1990, and it isn't effective now.

I refer to the next part as "brainwashing." Most people I've spoken to over the age of fifty, thousands of them, express similar concerns. They were all told to strengthen their leg muscles, lose weight, and keep moving. I call it brainwashing because this message is everywhere: on websites, in brochures, at doctors' offices, in personal training routines, and also told to us by physical therapists and nurses. Everyone is speaking the same language.

But let me share a few things that might genuinely surprise you.

I came across a Harvard newsletter that basically said, "We know your knee hurts, but keep moving anyway. That's the best thing you can do."[3] I remember thinking, *Whoever wrote this has clearly never felt real knee pain.* During my twenty years of pain, my knees were swollen, burning, and achy; being told to just "keep moving" felt almost cruel.

Then I read this from the Mayo Clinic: "Exercise helps ease arthritis pain and stiffness."[4]

And it hit me…

These messages all say the same thing: ignore your pain.

But here's what's wild: we were all raised to believe that if something hurts, you stop doing whatever is causing the pain. Yet we are repeatedly told the opposite by the Western medical industry: *keep going, push through, don't slow down.* For many people, following this advice leads not to healing but to further damage, particularly to the cartilage we are desperately trying to preserve.

I saw a heartbreaking comment recently from a woman online. She

---

[3.] Kelly Bilodeau, "Take Control of Your Knee Pain," *Harvard Health Publishing*, August 1, 2024, reviewed by Robert H. Shmerling, MD, Senior Faculty Editor, *Harvard Health Publishing*, https://www.health.harvard.edu/pain/take-control-of-your-knee-pain.

[4.] Mayo Clinic Staff, *Arthritis: Exercises that Help Ease Arthritis Pain and Stiffness*, Mayo Clinic, https://www.mayoclinic.org/diseases-conditions/arthritis/in-depth/arthritis/art-20047971. Mayo Clinic wrote, "I *fell in 2010. I've tried everything, even arthroscopic surgery—but the pain is unbearable. Now I'm on strong painkillers. What should I do?"*

Fifteen years of pain…

From one fall.

No answers.

Just stronger medications while inflammation slowly destroys her cartilage and damages her ligaments. Now she's facing the path many people eventually take.

From where I stand, the truth is starting to reveal itself… and it's not pretty.

The medical industry encourages over-the-counter drugs, such as Advil and Aleve. However, there's an important point they often over-look about these medications.

> **Knee Note:** *Adults and teens who are treating osteoarthritis may be directed by their healthcare provider to take 1,200 mg to 3,200 mg per day.*[5]

These drugs can damage your kidneys and liver. When you rely on them regularly to manage knee and hip pain, you may not be aware of the damage you're causing to your organs. Because these medications can mask pain, you might continue your normal activities without realizing that you are further harming your knees.

Using over-the-counter drugs can lead to kidney disease and liver disease at a young age. My client Diane is a perfect example of this. Though only forty-nine years old, she had been in pain for twenty years. Because she took over-the-counter drugs, she suffers from kidney disease. She was also on her way to getting double knee replacements.[6]

---

5. Arthritis Foundation, "Ibuprofen," Arthritis Foundation Drug Guide (Arthritis Foundation), last updated December 27, 2024, https://www.arthritis.org/drug-guide/nsaids/ibuprofen.
6. National Kidney Foundation, *Watch out for Your Kidneys When You Use Medicines for Pain*, News

Diane came to me with low expectations, having tried everything else without success. Despite her struggles, she trusted me and followed my advice closely. Doctors had told her they wouldn't perform the surgery because she was overweight, which added to her pain and sense of helplessness.

However, after working with me, Diane no longer needed knee replacement surgery. As of 2026, she still has her knees thanks to her commitment to my program and my step-by-step guidance. I am incredibly proud of her progress.

Now, let's talk about cortisone shots.

> **Knee Note:** *It's crucial to understand that **cortisone can damage cartilage**, making it more pliable and more prone to wear.[7] It's baffling that this treatment is recommended for knee pain when it actually quickens the deterioration in the cartilage.*

Now, I've heard many stories about cortisone injections. People often say, "It worked for one day," or "It worked for one week," but sometimes, they find that it doesn't work at all. In addition, injecting cortisone into your system can cause other health issues, such as raising blood sugar levels, if you're diabetic.

As I mentioned earlier, cortisone can have very different effects on the body; it either works or it doesn't. There's really no middle ground. What *is* unavoidable, however, is that cortisone injections tend to wear down your cartilage faster.

Doctors usually recommend no more than two to three cortisone shots per year. This number sounds scientific, but it's more of a polite guess than a hard rule.

Later in this book, I'll break down various treatment options, but for

---

& Stories, August 12, 2014, https://www.kidney.org/news-stories/watch-out-your-kidneys-when-you-use-medicines-pain.

7. Mayo Clinic Staff, *Cortisone Shots*, Mayo Clinic, last reviewed September 21, 2023, https://www.mayoclinic.org/tests-procedures/cortisone-shots/about/pac-20384794.

now, you should know that cortisone injections and over-the-counter medications are the two most common paths people are offered. Personally, I skipped both. Not because I enjoy suffering, but because I knew neither option was going to lead me to the other side of healing.

Now let's talk about the orthopedic model.

> **Knee Note:** *Remember, orthopedic doctors receive very limited training in pain management—often as little as eleven hours. As a result, their approach centers on rapid diagnosis and symptom control rather than long-term problem solving. This model has been passed down for decades and continues to shape how knee pain is treated today.*

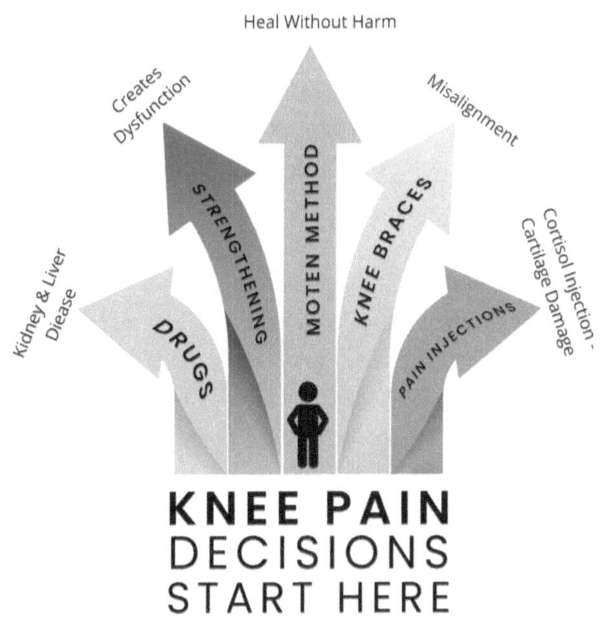

Looking at the diagram, which road would you choose?

When people visit an orthopedic specialist for knee pain or injury, they usually get a brief audition. When I saw four different doctors, my appointments averaged about fifteen minutes. They bent my knee, nodded thoughtfully, and prescribed physical therapy and anti-inflammatory drugs.

If your experience mirrors mine, they may also have casually mentioned cortisone, prolotherapy, or a Synvisc injection.

The orthopedic model often looks like this: you explain your knee problem, and they treat it the same way they treat *everyone else's*. The details don't matter much. The outcome is preselected.

You might leave with a shot, a prescription, or a referral to physical therapy, but very few questions are asked, especially the ones that matter. For example, *what other joints have started hurting since this began?* That question alone could change the entire conversation.

I've heard countless stories from clients who describe the same routine: a five-minute glance at their X-rays, followed by the dramatic reveal, "You have bone on bone." There's nothing you can do except manage the pain.

> ***Knee Note:*** *Bone-on-bone is considered an advanced stage of osteoarthritis; however, in some instances, it's just not true. There are numerous X-rays showing cartilage deterioration, but there is still cartilage between the two bones. If the person still has a meniscus, which is a cushion between the two bones, how is it possible for them to have bone-on-bone? We need to look at our X-rays and ask questions.*

What doctors often leave patients with is this advice: "When the pain becomes severe enough, come back for surgery." But this misses a crucial point: by offering no real hope and only the promise of future surgery, they overlook the very real consequences patients face, other joint problems, depression, weight gain, and a growing sense of hopelessness, just as I experienced.

Knee Note: Young athletes with knee and hip injuries face the possibility of developing PTOA (post-traumatic osteoarthritis) in later years if the orthopedic model is still prescribing PT, surgery, shots, and drugs as their only options.[8]

The longer we remain reliant on the orthopedic industry, the greater the risk of developing osteoarthritis and ultimately needing surgery. This industry focuses solely on managing pain rather than curing or healing.

I have often wondered why the same treatments I received in the 1990s are still being prescribed to patients today in 2026. Why has nothing changed?

In my research, I found that the orthopedic industry doesn't prioritize preventative care. They seem unconcerned about preventing issues like hip, back, or joint problems because they know they can't easily address these concerns. Instead, their focus is mainly on perfecting surgeries, as that's where the money lies.

I didn't want to admit this until I started seeing the numbers. By 2030, the demand for primary total hip arthroplasties is projected to increase by 174 percent to 572,000 procedures. The demand for primary total knee arthroplasties is projected to grow by 673 percent to 3.48 million procedures.[9]

The emphasis is on making total knee replacement surgeries more efficient and effective, often to the extent that some patients can go home the same day. According to the American Academy of Orthopedic Surgeons, from 2012 to 2024, there were over four million knee and hip replacements in the United States alone.[10]

---

8. Nicole A. Friel and Constance R. Chu, "The Role of ACL Injury in the Development of Posttraumatic Knee Osteoarthritis," *Clinical Sports Medicine* 32, no. 1 (January 2013): 1–12, https://www.ncbi.nlm.nih.gov/pmc/articles/PMC6548436/.

9. Steven Kurtz, Kevin Ong, Edmund Lau, Fionna Mowat, and Michael Halpern, "Projections of Primary and Revision Hip and Knee Arthroplasty in the United States from 2005 to 2030," *The Journal of Bone and Joint Surgery, American Volume* 89, no. 4 (April 2007): 780–85, https://pubmed.ncbi.nlm.nih.gov/17403800/.

10. American Academy of Orthopaedic Surgeons, "American Joint Replacement Registry Marks

I have noticed that many professionals in this field quietly steer patients toward robotic surgeries, often with very little discussion about alternatives. This fifteen-billion-dollar industry frequently runs on pain, fear, and a lack of patient education rather than truly comprehensive care.

What concerns me most is that I do not believe many doctors fully recognize the long-term consequences of this approach, especially their resistance to prevention and alternative solutions. It is as if the idea of stopping pain before it escalates is somehow more radical than replacing a joint.

At one point, I reached out to the Arthritis Association because I genuinely believed they would want to hear a different perspective. I wanted to show them how effective my methods were for me and for others. Their response was polite but dismissive. They told me, "Renee, we have so many people coming to us with ideas. We have to pick and choose which ones we address."

At that moment, I thought, if people are actually getting better, would that not be worth at least a second look?

I have X-rays from 2004, 2011, and 2021 that clearly show osteoarthritis. What is missing from that timeline is deterioration. My condition is not getting worse. That detail, however, does not seem to fit neatly into the current narrative, so it is conveniently ignored. The possibility that something could change the entire industry and help people live without constant pain appears to make some very uncomfortable.

I also applied for a grant from the Arthritis Association, thinking that if funding entered the picture, curiosity might follow. It turns out the Arthritis Association does not provide grants to holistic practitioners. Which is puzzling to me, considering Western medicine has been trying to find a solution since the 1700s.

The word "arthritis" dates back to the 1700s, and the condition itself

---

Record Growth, Strengthens Global Collaboration," press release, October 23, 2025, https://www.aaos.org/aaos-home//newsroom/press-releases/ajrr-annual-report-press-release/. AAOS was recognized long before that. Centuries later, arthritis is still here, and effective pain relief remains elusive. Visit any arthritis-related website, and you will quickly be asked to donate. The question is why. What research is being funded, and why does the outcome never seem to change?

The real reason doctors have not found a way to stop osteoarthritis from progressing is not a lack of effort. It is that they are looking in the wrong places.

Painkillers

How many joints need to hurt before doctors acknowledge that their methods aren't effective? No matter how many times you visit the doctor with issues in your knees, hips, or back, they tend to provide the same misguided advice. When they start discussing treatment options, the conversation often begins with suggestions to lose weight and strengthen weak leg muscles, followed by a discussion of injections.

Let's take a closer look at these injections and other pain-management options available for knee problems. There are several types:

1. **Corticosteroids (cortisone)**: While they can provide temporary relief, they can also damage your cartilage.
2. **Hyaluronic acid (Synvisc)** injections: These are intended to lubricate your joints, but they usually last no more than three months and do not heal your knees.
3. **Platelet-rich plasma (PRP) therapy**: This method shows some promise, as it involves injecting your own platelet-rich plasma into the knee. While it may provide longer-lasting relief than other injections, it remains a temporary solution.
4. **Stem cell therapy:** Needs good blood flow; this is critical for stem cell therapy. Knee cartilage is avascular, meaning it lacks its own blood vessels. Poor circulation in the joint can lead to a toxic environment that prevents these cells from surviving or differentiating into new cartilage.

Now, let's discuss supplements. We are often advised to take glucosamine. In my view, glucosamine can be dangerous. It lubricates the joints, but it can mask pain for years, leading people to underestimate their condition. I have seen at least three clients who experienced pain for seven to ten years. Because they were on glucosamine, they didn't realize the extent of their pain, resulting in damage to their ligaments. Once ligaments are damaged, the knee can start to bow, ultimately requiring surgery. I do not recommend glucosamine at all.

Regarding physical therapy, it's important to note that their treatment is typically dictated by doctors. No matter the specific issue with your knee, doctors often prescribe the same basic exercises, limiting the therapist's ability to tailor treatment to individual needs.

For instance, my client's right knee, lower back, and left hip were hurting. She also experienced shoulder tightness, neck aches, and her knees waking her at night.

> ***Knee Note:*** *Please note this is how people with chronic knee pain enter into physical therapy. They come with many other joint issues.*

However, when she went to physical therapy, the focus was usually only on her knee. This approach did little to address her other joint problems, which were exacerbated by the orthopedic industry's tendency to simply manage pain rather than solve underlying issues.

Physical therapists often concentrate on one area of the body, neglecting the patient's neck, back, and hip pain, which means the root problems remain unresolved. As a result, they risk developing more osteoarthritis in other joints and undergoing more surgery in the future. **Will someone in the medical industry please listen?**

Creams and ointments may provide temporary relief, perhaps by warming up the knee, but they do not heal anything.

Weight loss is often suggested as a solution. I lost 25 pounds and saw no change. The issue is not merely about weight or the amount of load; rather, it's about dysfunction in the rest of the body.

Orthotics. If your podiatrist takes a mold of your foot to suggest orthotics, your question should be, "Why do I need them? What has changed in my foot that requires an orthotic?" I was fitted with orthotics because I have plantar fasciitis. My next question should've been, "Why do I have plantar fasciitis?" We have to get to the root cause of our pain and not allow doctors to give us temporary fixes.

Surgical interventions, such as arthroscopic surgery, frequently result in scar tissue, which can lead to additional problems.

We need a paradigm shift in how we approach joint health. I encourage you to embrace a new way of thinking, one that moves beyond outdated eighteenth-century approaches and toward more effective healing solutions. As I mentioned earlier, the orthopedic industry, shaped by its traditional training, often focuses on immediate diagnosis and symptom management through medication.

We all want to make the best decisions for our joint health. The challenge is that we are rarely given the full story. We trust the people in white coats and accept their solutions without question. Here's what the orthopedic industry typically recommends:

- Prescribe medication
- Strengthening around your inflamed knee
- Wearing a knee brace
- Cortisone shots
- Physical Therapy
- Injections
- Over-the-counter drugs

All of these will eventually lead to osteoarthritis and then surgery. Why? Because they only manage the pain while your knee continues to deteriorate, and your hip and back start to hurt. This is just not right.

My solution, The Knee Pain Recipe, is combined with The Moten Method, which only uses holistic methods to reduce your inflammation and swelling and create an extraordinary healing environment. You will learn more about the recipe in later chapters.

3

WHY KNEE REPLACEMENT IS SO COMMON

One reason total knee replacement (TKR) has become so common is that people are told what is happening inside their knee, but not *why* it happened. Knee arthritis is not a life sentence, and it is not an automatic path to total knee replacement (TKR). We are no longer in an era of limited understanding.

In 2026, knowledge and education give us the power to interrupt the cycle that leads so many people straight to surgery. In this book, I will show you why total knee replacement is approaching the end of its era. Medical history reminds us that many conditions once treated with drastic interventions eventually became manageable or even preventable through better understanding.

Just as the management of HIV and polio was transformed by targeting their biological origins, knee care is entering a new era of understanding. By applying the science behind the kinetic chain and how our overall health affects our knees, we can now treat the actual cause of knee wear and tear instead of just hiding the pain.

So if you need surgery, here are a few things to consider. When someone undergoes total knee replacement (TKR) surgery, they may not be informed about the risks of nerve damage, drop foot, calf and shin pain, or potential allergic reactions to the metal used in the knee implant or even the bandages.

> **Knee Note:** *Before going into surgery, ask what type of metal they are going to use for the surgery. Check to see if you are allergic to the bandages.*

I recently heard from a woman on my social media page who said she wished she had never undergone knee replacement surgery. Despite having both knees replaced, she continues to live with pain five years later.

This is why I urge people to preserve their natural knees for as long as possible. A total knee replacement is irreversible. Once bone is shaved and surrounding muscles and ligaments are disrupted, the outcomes can vary widely. Some people do very well. Others discover that "fixed" does not always mean "comfortable," and that the story does not always end happily ever after.

Once complications set in, there is very little anyone can do unless another surgery is added to the plan. And once you start down that road, it tends to stay under construction. So hold on to your knees for as long as you can. The consequences of staying locked into the orthopedic system can be life-altering. You may find yourself becoming dependent on family members. A spouse can slowly shift from partner to caretaker. Children may feel the quiet pressure of needing to help because getting up and moving is no longer simple or spontaneous.

Vacations begin to revolve around knees instead of destinations. Trips are planned with questions that never used to matter. Are there stairs? How far is the walk? Will the chairs be forgiving enough to sit down and get back up without turning it into a group activity? These calculations weigh heavily on people with knee pain, often long before the trip even begins.

And life should not require this much planning just to go on vacation.

Knee Note: In 2019, about 528 million people worldwide were living with osteoarthritis, an increase of 113 percent since 1990.

Global Impact and Prevalence

- Knee osteoarthritis (KOA) is a major global health issue, with an alarming increase in cases, prevalence, and disability-adjusted life years (DALYs) since 1990.
- It is the leading cause of disability globally.
- In 2020, the global prevalence was 7.96 percent of the population, and the number of years lived with disability due to all osteoarthritis rose by 9.5 percent from 1990 to 2020.
- In the US, around one in seven adults has OA, and it is the most common cause of disability.[1]

When you go shopping, you need to think about how far you can walk from the store to your car. A cart becomes essential for support as you shop.

If you have to do your own laundry, you may need to navigate stairs with a laundry basket, which poses a risk of falling.

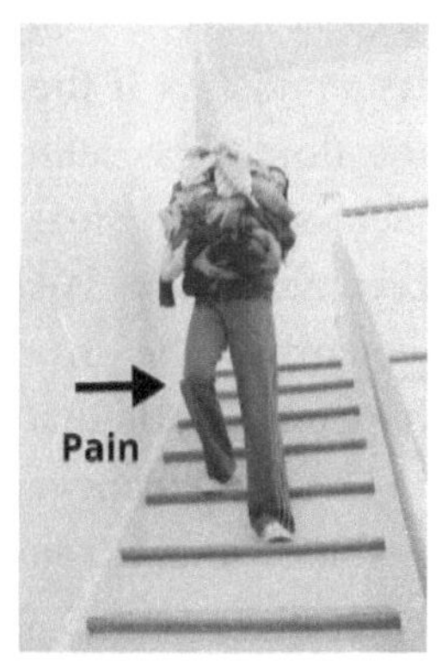

Many people are moving out of their homes simply because they have stairs that they can no longer manage.

Moreover, a lot of people feel like they are becoming a burden. I remember a woman who felt she had to go on vacation; she wanted to spend time with her daughter, but she worried that her knee problems would prevent her from enjoying herself. This pain doesn't just affect the individual; it impacts the whole family.

---

1. Y. Ouyang *et al.*, "Global, Regional, and National Burden of Knee Osteoarthritis," *Journal of Orthopaedic Surgery and Research* (2025), https://www.ncbi.nlm.nih.gov/pmc/articles/PMC12351899/. PMC

Here in the United States, we do not need to wait to get TKR. In other countries, like Canada, the situation can be even more challenging.[2]

I have a client from Canada who has severe osteoarthritis and has been in pain for about five years. Her knees remain swollen, and she faces an additional challenge: she is a caretaker. Imagine juggling that responsibility while dealing with knee problems. For her, securing an appointment with an orthopedist could take up to two years before she can get her TKR. This is one of the reasons why I receive messages from all over the world, from Germany, Nigeria, Italy, India, and many other countries, asking, sometimes begging, for help.

To gain access to the necessary medical evaluations, you first have to see the specialist. After the evaluation, if the doctor determines that surgery is needed, there is often a two-year waiting list for the procedure in Canada. This is where significant consequences arise.

While waiting for surgery, patients continue to walk on their affected joints, which exacerbates deterioration. Swelling is one of the biggest reasons why ligament damage occurs. It's almost as if the ligament is drowning in the fluid. The cellular structure of the ligament starts to break down, and the ligament becomes weak. Weak ligaments in the knee jeopardize the integrity of the knee. What happens next is that the knee will bow, either in or out. Whichever way it is doesn't matter because you will need surgery in the future, regardless.

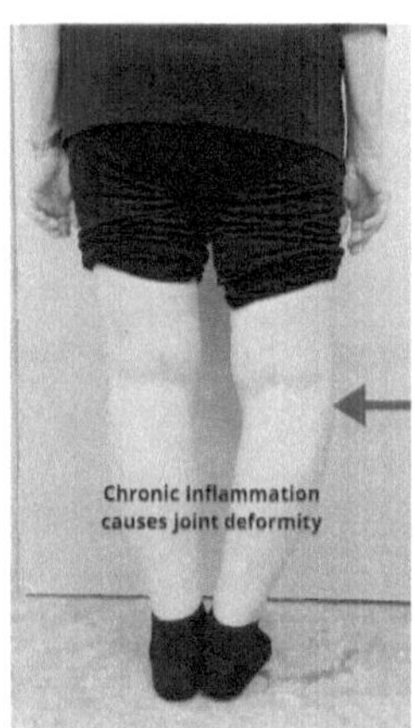

Knee Note: When you're on a waiting list, that means increased cartilage damage. This delay can create an imbalance in the whole body,

---

2. Amina Zafar, "It's Much Faster to Get Hip or Knee Replacements if There's a Central Waitlist: Study," *CBC News*, May 20, 2025, https://www.cbc.ca/news/health/hip-knee-replacement-waits-faster-1.7537443. Novari Health

which will affect the hips and the back. More surgeries will be needed in the future.

In this scenario, the patient must wait two years for knee surgery. Once they finally undergo the procedure, their knee may be fixed, but what about the hip pain? What about their back? It's possible that their other knee has also begun to hurt. Unfortunately, the surgery only addresses the one knee, leaving other issues unresolved.

As people continue to walk this path, the pain rarely stays put. The hip joins the conversation, the back chimes in, and sometimes the other knee decides it would also like attention. One replacement quietly leads to another, and before long, the hip knows its turn is next. The real issue, overall musculoskeletal health, was never addressed. Instead, one knee gets a temporary fix while the rest of the body struggles to compensate.

This is how people end up needing additional knee replacements and, in some cases, hip replacements as well. These outcomes are not bad luck. They are the predictable result of an industry that treats parts instead of people. For those diagnosed with osteoarthritis, it can feel like the future has already been decided.

As I mentioned earlier, once you have one knee replacement, there is almost a ninety percent chance you will need another. Injections are not a long-term solution. They are more like a pause button. Helpful for a moment, but the pain resumes right where it left off. Most injections do not truly reduce inflammation, and they certainly do not reverse damage or correct dysfunctional movement patterns. They simply buy time, often at a very high cost.

Many people stay stuck in this cycle because that is what they are told to do. Follow the plan. Come back in six months. Try another shot. Repeat as needed.

Dear reader, I'm not here to rewrite the medical textbook. I just want you to be aware that while your doctor's 'toolbox' is vital for emergencies, it is often limited to drugs, shots, and surgery when it comes to chronic knee pain. You deserve to know about the alternatives that exist outside of your doctor's office.

> ***Knee Note:*** *There is some promise in the Western medicine world. I have seen articles in which The University of Utah has begun to examine people's gait and found that this may be a contributing factor to the pain levels of OA.*[3] *This is good news.*

---

3. Lerner, Evan. "New Study Shows Gait Retraining Could Significantly Reduce Knee Pain from Osteoarthritis and Potentially Slow Cartilage Damage." *The John and Marcia Price College of Engineering at the University of Utah*, 12 Aug. 2025, www.price.utah.edu/2025/08/12/new-study-shows-gait-retraining-could-significantly-reduce-knee-pain-from-osteoarthritis-and-potentially-slow-cartilage-damage.

4

KINETIC CHAIN RESTORING JOINT HARMONY

What is a kinetic chain? Your body does not work in isolated parts. It works as a chain. Every step you take sends force from the ground up through your foot, ankle, knee, hip, and shoulder. This sequence is called the **kinetic chain**. When each link moves in harmony with the others, the force is absorbed and distributed smoothly. But when one link is

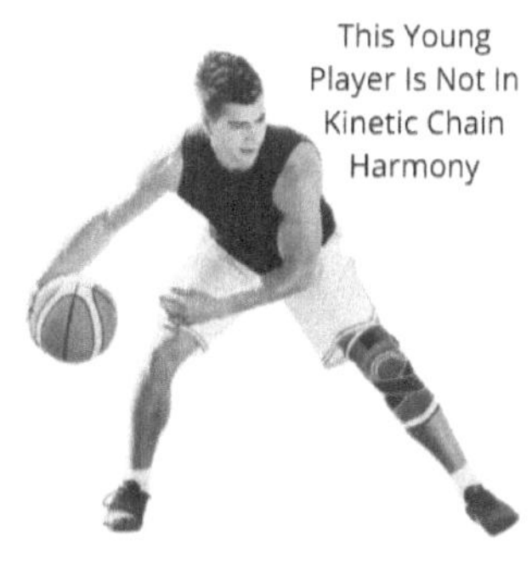

This Young Player Is Not In Kinetic Chain Harmony

restricted or weak, or an injury occurs, this creates a misalignment. The body adapts by compensating elsewhere. Over time, those compensations create limping, muscle imbalance, joint stress, and eventually chronic pain. The knee is rarely the starting point; it's simply where the breakdown becomes impossible to ignore.

Knee Note: The NIH Library of Medicine states, "Knee osteoarthritis is associated with increased movement at the ankle joint; attention should be paid to the ankle joint when treating patients with knee osteoarthritis."[1]

This single sentence quietly exposes why so many knee treatments fail. Chronic knee pain is not just a knee problem; it is a kinetic chain problem. When the ankle is forced to absorb an abnormal load, the knee pays the price. To correct the imbalance and stop the cycle of pain, we must stop chasing the knee and start where movement begins: the ankles.

An imbalance in the kinetic chain is what keeps us in pain for one, five, or ten years, and sometimes even more. So, what really causes this imbalance, and how do you correct it?

Through all my research and lived experience, I've discovered something surprising: it isn't just the pain itself that keeps us stuck; it's the misconceptions surrounding it. There are **four major lies (myths)** we've been taught to believe, and they quietly prolong our suffering.

Myth #1: "Your pain is caused by being overweight."

I'm sure you've heard this one; I certainly have. My doctor told me to strengthen my leg muscles and lose weight. I wasn't exactly heavy, but I dutifully lost twenty-five pounds anyway, thinking, *This is it! My knees will finally behave!* I looked amazing... but my knees were still screaming. Apparently, my knees didn't get the memo.

Myth #2: "Just keep moving and exercising."

It's everywhere: *Move, move, move!* Supposedly, it keeps your joints happy and lubricated. And yes, sometimes you wake up stiff, take a few steps, and feel a tiny bit better.

Here's the kicker: every step with misaligned joints can actually wear down your cartilage faster. Surprise! Not exactly what they told you on the website.

---

[1] Du Hyun Ro, Joonhee Lee, Jangyun Lee, Jae-Young Park, Hyuk-Soo Han, and Myung Chul Lee, "Effects of Knee Osteoarthritis on Hip and Ankle Gait Mechanics," *Advances in Orthopedics* 2019 (2019), https://www.ncbi.nlm.nih.gov/pmc/articles/PMC6451827/.

I know what you are thinking: *So if I don't move, I'll stiffen up?* Don't worry. I've got you; I'll show you how to move without wrecking your knees.

Myth #3: "Strengthen your leg muscles to take pressure off your knees."

Whoever came up with this advice clearly never had knee pain. You're telling me to strengthen sore, inflamed, stiff knees, and somehow that's supposed to help? Traditional strengthening exercises often make the pain worse, not better, because they ignore the real issue: faulty movement patterns, inflammation, and misalignment.

Myth #4: "Pain is just a natural part of aging."

I hear this myth all the time: "I'm in pain because I'm getting old."

Who decided that turning seventy, eighty, or ninety means you must live in pain? And what does that mean for the millions of people suffering in their forties, fifties, and sixties? Their pain isn't caused by age, and neither is yours. Weight, movement, and age are not the root issues. Something else is happening. Read on

We are in pain because we're all following the same script handed down by the orthopedic industry. Unless we change how we think about our bodies and our pain, we will continue to suffer.

A comment on my social media touched my heart. A woman wrote, *"I am currently bone on bone in my knee, and walking is impossible. My other knee and hip hurt too, and there's no cartilage left. Now I've been told I need a knee replacement. I am in total shock; this is so traumatic for me."*

Her story is not rare. It reflects a painful truth: people do everything they're told, yet they're still in agony. This is why we must rethink the entire narrative around pain and recovery.

I hear stories like this every single day: people who "did everything right." They listened to their doctors. They trusted their physical therapists. They pushed through the pain because they were told that healing required discomfort. Yet healing never came. In fact, the pain got worse.

Another woman commented on my social media platform: *"I lost weight. I stretched. I walked. I even had arthroscopic surgery three months ago… and I'm still in pain."*

How does this happen? How can someone lose weight, exercise, and have surgery, only to end up in more pain than before? Meanwhile, the solution offered is always the same: another appointment, another medication, another injection, or a surgeon standing by, sometimes with a robot ready to operate.

So why do we stay in pain? Hold on. I am getting to the answer. Healing is not only about what you do with your body. It is also about how you think.

One major reason people remain stuck is what I call the orthopedic trap.

Take knee braces, for example. They are often one of the first things a doctor recommends. And I understand the appeal. When your knee hurts, you naturally want support. As of 2026, the global knee braces market is estimated at approximately \$2.74 billion.[2]

But let's be honest. How many of you have worn one of those braces with the hole cut out over the kneecap? They may feel helpful at first, but they do not actually stabilize the kneecap. In many cases, they do the opposite. Relying on them can create new problems because the body is designed to move as a balanced system. When one area is braced and doing less work, another area is forced to work harder to compensate.

And compensation is often where the real trouble begins.

The only time I recommend wearing a knee brace is after surgery or during an acute injury that truly requires temporary stabilization.

---

[2] Lexixf Solutions. 2025. "Knee Brace Market Installed Base Expansion & Outlook 2026-2033." *LinkedIn*, December 30, 2025. The global knee brace market was valued at approximately USD 2.5 billion in 2023 and is projected to grow at a CAGR of about 6.8% from 2024 to 2030, reaching an estimated USD 4.4 billion by the end of the forecast period. https://www.linkedin.com/pulse/knee-brace-market-installed-base-expansion-outlook-2026-2033-n9ftc/.

Wearing a brace while running, exercising, or even walking is counterproductive; it can actually push you closer to surgery. A brace will not make you more active, but it forces your body to work harder in the wrong ways.

This message came into my chat box recently: *"Please help me. I have a meniscus tear in my left knee and osteoarthritis in both knees. I had knee surgery, and my knee still hurts ten years later."*

Stories like this are incredibly common. Knee surgery does not guarantee miraculous or immediate relief. In fact, about 30 percent of people continue to have issues afterward.[3] There is a reason why chronic pain persists and why so many eventually need another surgery.

How many joints have to hurt before doctors admit their methods aren't working? You can walk into the office with knee, hip, or back pain, and the advice rarely changes.

This is exactly where I come in.

I understand why people continue to suffer, why pain persists, and why so many need additional knee or hip replacements. The root cause has been ignored, and I discovered it. That's why I am now pain-free. I have osteoarthritis in both knees and hips, yet I am very functional for someone who has had twenty years of pain. I can walk long distances, jump rope, climb mountains, and hike, all because I found the root cause of my pain.[4]

Now let's shift gears, because this is the part that actually changes everything.

After years of research, relentless observation, and thousands of real bodies standing right in front of me, I uncovered what most people are

---

[3]. Xiaoying Wang, Mitsuru Ida, Kayo Uyama, Yusuke Naito, and Masahiko Kawaguchi, "Persistent Postoperative Pain at 1 Year after Orthopedic Surgery and Its Association with Functional Disability," *Journal of Anesthesia* 37, no. 2 (2023): 248–53, https://pubmed.ncbi.nlm.nih.gov/36565365/. pubmed.ncbi.nlm.nih.gov.

[4]. https://youtube.com/shorts/pTfchsnLS7E?feature=share.

never told about chronic knee pain. And yes, it surprises almost everyone who hears it.

Chronic knee pain is not caused by age. It is not caused by weight, weak knees, or some inevitable "wear and tear" story we have been taught to accept. The real cause is a full-body imbalance created by **limping**.

Yes, limping. For some people, that imbalance begins quietly with the development of a bunion on the big toe. Then into an improper walking gait, and then knee pain.

For others, the problem starts much earlier. On the court. On the field. In Zumba classes. Sports like tennis, golf, basketball, and baseball naturally create dominance on one side of the body. Without intentional rebalancing, that dominance slowly transfers stress into the knees and hips.

Over time, this imbalance reshapes the way you walk, run, and load your body. The knee, caught in the middle, becomes the casualty.

It may sound almost too simple. But stay with me, because this is where everything begins to make sense.

During my struggle, people would constantly ask, "Renee, why are you limping?" and I would insist I wasn't. I truly believed I wasn't. But everything changed the day I looked at the soles of my shoes and noticed uneven wear. Specifically, the bottom of my right shoe had worn down, creating an actual hole.

That was the moment I realized something was off on my right side, but I didn't fully grasp how serious it was.

When we limp, our entire body becomes dysfunctional. We fall out of balance. One side grows stronger and overworked, while the other gets weaker. Then we take that imbalanced body up and down stairs. We play sports. We jog, walk, and perform strengthening exercises, and then wonder why our joints are still hurting. Before long, the opposite knee starts to hurt… then the hip… then the lower back. Limping causes a cascading effect.

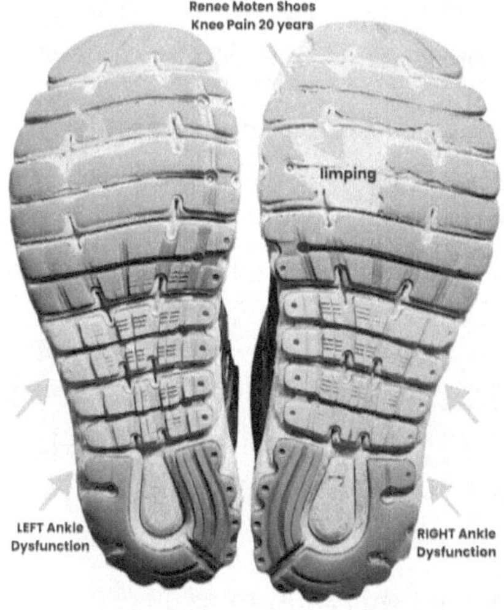

Knee pain causes limping. Shoe wear proves it.

Limping stresses a healthy joint in an unnatural way until it becomes painful. This is often the *root cause* of why we got into pain in the first place and the very reason we can't seem to get out of it. Until we acknowledge that one side of the body is stronger than the other, true healing can't begin.

If you play sports or exercise, you're constantly aware of that "bad knee." But that hyper-awareness creates even more imbalance. And imbalance doesn't stay in one place; it spreads. It can lead to back spasms, rotator cuff injuries, plantar fasciitis, foot and leg cramps, and even a stiff neck.

After three to six months of pain that comes and goes, it's now classi-fied as chronic. At that point, the limp has set in, and it begins affecting your entire body.

So, how do we get back into balance?

How do we break the cycle of dysfunction?

I'm ready to introduce you to my secret weapon.

Do you have a pen handy?

The secret weapon is understanding the **kinetic chain**, the ultimate joint protector in most traditional treatments for joint dysfunction.

Think about it: gymnasts and ballet dancers live by the kinetic chain. Their upper and lower body must move in perfect harmony to perform at the elite level their craft demands. When you apply these same principles to knee pain, mobility, and alignment, you can become just as unstoppable.

Most people dealing with knee injuries, ankle issues, osteoarthritis, or hip, back, and neck pain don't realize they've put stress on their entire kinetic chain. Once this chain is disrupted, healing and rebalancing are essential.

If you don't understand this concept and ignore your pain, you begin to "break" the chain link by link. The longer inflammation and swelling remain, the more links fail, and the more dysfunction you'll experience throughout your body.

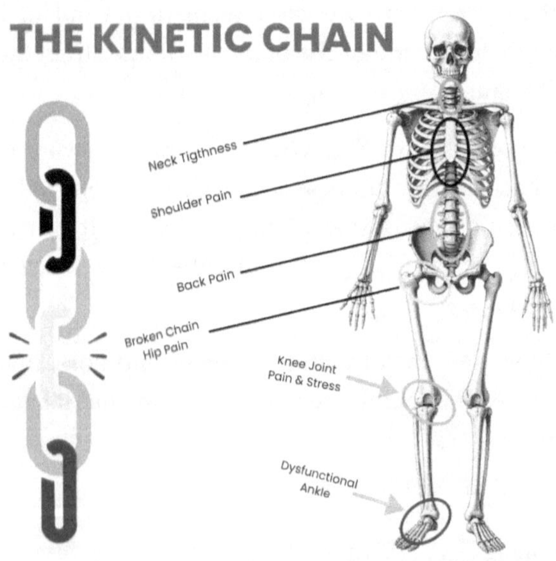

Persistent knee pain leads to limping. **Limping breaks the kinetic chain.**

This image shows how hip pain affects everything: neck tightness, shoulder and back pain, knee pain, and even a dysfunctional ankle. **This is the power of the kinetic chain, and why restoring balance is a critical key to lasting pain reduction.**

Persistent pain or recurring injuries can be frustrating, especially when conventional treatments only address the site of discomfort without providing a lasting solution.

As we move into 2026, I invite you to embrace a new way of thinking about your health, one that breaks free from the limited educational abilities of the orthopedic doctors. It's time to think differently, move differently, and finally reclaim the pain-free life you deserve.

Knee Note: Food for Thought

An estimated 528 million people worldwide are currently living with osteoarthritis.[5] Projections show that knee osteoarthritis alone is expected to double by 2050, contributing to nearly 1 billion OA cases globally. The knee brace market is projected to reach $4.4 billion by 2030, and total knee replacements have increased by 188% among adults ages 45–64.[6,7]

These trends are not signs of progress — they are warning signals

---

5. World Health Organization. *Osteoarthritis.* Fact sheet, July 14, 2023. https://www.who.int/news-room/fact-sheets/detail/osteoarthritis.

6. Lexixf Solutions, *"Knee Brace Market Installed Base Expansion & Outlook 2026-2033,"* LinkedIn, published December 30, 2025, global knee brace market valued at approximately USD 2.5 billion in 2023 and projected to grow significantly by 2030.

7. Arthritis Foundation, *"The Risks of Early Knee Replacement Surgery,"* Arthritis Foundation, published 2025, article on rising revision surgeries and long-term risks of early knee replacement, https://www.arthritis.org/health-wellness/treatment/joint-surgery/safety-and-risks/the-risks-of-early-knee-replacement-surgery.

5

SIGNS YOUR BODY'S OFF BALANCE

For years, conventional medicine has trained us to see knee pain through a very small, very busy window: take this pill, get this shot, and if all else fails, surprise! Here comes surgery. It's a greatest-hits playlist of quick fixes, all designed to quiet the pain and shove us back into motion as fast as possible, whether our bodies are actually ready or not.

And sure, sometimes it works… briefly. The problem never truly went away because the knee was treated like an independent contractor, not part of a full-body system with rules, relationships, and consequences.

This book is an invitation to stop slapping temporary patches on a deeper problem. This thinking requires a paradigm shift. And no, that's not a trendy buzzword. A paradigm shift simply means learning something new, questioning what you've been told, and being willing to look at your situation through a different lens, preferably one that isn't fogged up by years of frustration.

WHICH PATH WOULD YOU CHOOSE?

PARADIGM SHIFT

DOCTORS VISIT

Strengthen muscles → Wear a knee brace / Keep moving → Cortisone Shot

Lose weight → Physical Therapy → Anti-inflammatory drugs

Osteoarthritis / Total Knee Replacement Surgery

THE MOTEN METHOD

Gait Anaysis → Reduce Inflammation → Flexibility Alignment

Ankle Assessment → Reduce Swelling & Toxicty → Stability and Strengthening

Climb stair / Exercise/Play sports / Walk/Jog / Freedom from Pain

I had to make that shift myself. When you live with constant pain, curiosity becomes survival. You start asking, *What else is out there? Why isn't this working? There has to be another way.* In this chapter, I invite you to do the same. Open the door to a new way of thinking. Look at your knee pain differently. Let this be the moment you stop settling and start considering what's actually possible.

I want to share what is available in 2026 that can make a difference for all of us. I have devoted twenty-four years to researching just one area: the knees.

Ten of those years were just trying to figure out how to get out of pain. These last fourteen years have been about how to stay out of pain and create the proper exercises to complement my method.

Why focus on knees for twenty-four years? Simple: I spent years in pain with both knees, and then my hips decided to join the party. And all of it came from following outdated medical advice. (You know... the same advice many of us have been told for decades.)

In this chapter, my goal is to help you take a vacation without fear, drive long distances without stiffness, and get back to the game you love. I want you to feel like *yourself* again, and trust me, that transformation is possible with what I'm about to share.

So, let's dive in. Keep an open mind as we take this paradigm shift together. If you're still with me, raise your hand… Yes, I can see you.

Let's talk about the early warning signs of dysfunction: the little signals your body gives you when things are starting to shift out of balance. You might be surprised: corns, calluses, bunions, plantar fasciitis, orthotics, and that annoying ankle weakness after an injury. All of these are red flags that your kinetic chain is under stress. Remember: your foundation is your feet, ankles, calves, and shins.

Other warning signs come from activity-specific pain. You know the lines:

"I only have pain when I perform lunges or squats."

"I only have pain when I jog."

"I only have stiffness when I get out of bed."

"I only have pain when I go down the stairs."

This is a trap. The pain is easy to dismiss because it's "not that bad." Many women tell me, "I have a high pain tolerance," or "Knee pain isn't going to stop me," or "It only hurts every now and then." I have watched men and women whose knee pain is so severe that every step makes them limp, compensate, and shift their weight with each movement. This mindset, pushing through pain instead of understanding it, quietly accelerates joint breakdown. Pain that appears occasionally does not stay occasional. Over time, it becomes constant. What begins as something you tolerate can steadily move you closer and closer to a total knee replacement.

> ***Knee Note:*** *Asking for help when we're in pain isn't a weakness; it's wisdom. Especially for women, who are often taught to put everyone's needs first.*

You need your feet, ankles, shins, and calves to function well. That's your foundation. If the foundation is off, everything above it (the knees, hips, back, and neck) starts paying the price.

Other signs you're out of alignment? Constant tight calves and hamstrings, endless foam rolling on the IT band, and a stiff back every time you stand up. These are warning signals, not inconveniences; do not ignore them. This is exactly why I created the Knee Pain Reduction Strap (which I'll introduce in a later chapter): a tool that helps realign the kinetic chain without complicated exercises or guesswork.

> *Here's a quick tip: my "Knee Keeper Hint": restoring balance is essential for relieving pain. The Knee Pain Reduction Strap helps you achieve proper alignment without constantly trying to remember how to move correctly. It supports the process so you can get back to walking your dog, shopping without pain, and waking up in the morning without feeling like your joints are rusted shut.*

In the previous chapter, you saw an image of a hole in the bottom of my right shoe. That hole was from dragging my right leg after an ankle injury from soccer. I went to four doctors, seven chiropractors, six acupuncturists, and fifty-five massage therapists, yet not one of them asked to see my shoes. If they had, they would've spotted the wear pattern immediately, and maybe I would not be writing this book.

A hole in your shoe means everything is affected: knees, hips, shoulders, you name it. Yet the medical and fitness industries rarely consider footwear. This is a huge missed opportunity.

Before starting a walking or jogging program, you must undergo a **gait analysis**. The wear patterns on your shoes reveal the story of your gait. If you're dealing with knee issues, bring your shoes to your orthopedic surgeon. They might not look at them, but *you* should. Shoes don't lie.

These are the warning signs that your social world is getting smaller. You know the lines:

"I used to play pickleball."

"I used to practice yoga."

"I used to play basketball."

"I used to exercise four times a week… but now I can't."

It's important to understand that the knee joint is one of the largest and one of the strongest joints in the entire body. It's built like a tank. So, if *that* joint starts hurting? That knee has been under stress for months, sometimes even years.

This is where I need you to shift your thinking.

After I hurt my ankle playing soccer, things slowly spiraled. First, my feet started hurting months after the injury. Then came plantar fasciitis two years after the injury. Then I started limping. Five years later, my knee finally started yelling at me. Five years! My knee had been taking abuse quietly in the background the whole time, but because it didn't hurt yet, I had no clue anything was wrong.

So, when your knee finally starts hurting, it's not a "new" problem. It's an old issue that has finally reached its limit. And if you ignore it? It will gladly pass the stress on to other joints. Misery loves company.

This is where my approach differs from many medical professionals.

When you walk into a doctor's office with a knee problem or injury, the default plan is often the same: MRIs and X-rays, followed by drugs, injections, surgery, a brace, or physical therapy. Then the managed treatment of pain begins.

When you come to me with a knee problem or injury, I start differently. Yes, I review your doctor's report, but I don't jump straight to treating the knee. I watch you walk. I assess your gait. I look at the bottom of your shoes. I ask questions about your feet, your hips, your back, and any other joint pain you may have.

Only then do we begin a holistic journey to reduce inflammation and swelling, because I know what's *really* happening.

And one more thing: never ignore that **"little pain."**

It isn't little.

It's a warning flare.

After years of limping and being out of balance, the arches start to collapse. That's when your podiatrist suggests orthotics. Not because your feet suddenly "went bad," but because you became out of balance. The orthotics are trying to correct a deeper problem: your kinetic chain has been off for a long time.

And that's what I'm here to fix.

In this image, the body is out of balance. Millions of people are trying to strengthen their bodies when they're out of balance. **This imbalance is where chronic pain comes from**.

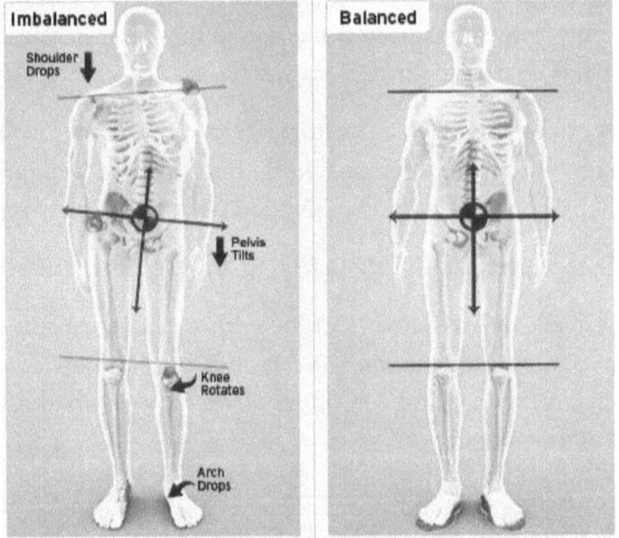

It's important to see your body as a whole, not as a collection of lonely body parts trying to figure life out on their own. One of my favorite tips for protecting your knees is this: meniscus tears don't usually happen out of nowhere. You might hear a pop and think, *All I did was turn around! I didn't do CrossFit, didn't climb a mountain, didn't run a marathon. I just... turned.*

But trust me, that one turn was a mountain and a culprit. That was just the final straw after years of stress your knee had been silently dealing with.

Most of the time, meniscus tears happen because the knee has been working overtime: twisting, turning, and pivoting during Zumba, basketball, tennis, or just living your best life. Then, one day… pop. Your knee finally files a complaint.

> **Knee Note:** *Zumba participants should ONLY be taught on smooth, even surfaces. No cracks, no bumps, no crooked tiles. And the shoes? It is a wise suggestion to* wear shoes recommended for Zumba Class. *You need shoes made for twisting. Wooden floors and basketball courts are the best surfaces.*

When it comes to knee pain, I don't believe most of it is "temporary." If you've got pain, you need to address it *immediately*. I know someone who simply stepped out of his car, turned his knee, and boom, two years of pain. Not because the injury was bad, but because he was given the wrong treatment.

As for me? I never injured my knee… Yet I lived with knee pain for twenty years. Why? Because of the orthopedic industry.

Let's talk about the warning signs of a misaligned kinetic chain.

If we understood how our bodies work internally, we'd see that every joint is connected, literally. Muscles, tendons, and joints communicate like co-workers on a group chat. You move one joint? The whole crew gets the memo.

So, how does the kinetic chain get out of whack?

- Joint Injuries
- Limping or compensating
- Foot issues (corns, calluses, bunions)
- Losing flexibility
- And the biggest culprit… sitting. Yes, sitting!

Let's talk about that last one because it's sneaky.

Every time you sit, your psoas (a muscle in the front of your hip) shortens. Sit long enough, and when you stand, you feel that urge to stretch your back. If that becomes a habit, congratulations. You're officially misaligned. Don't ignore that stiffness. It can turn into chronic hip or back pain.

If you drive for a living? Same problem. Hours of sitting lead to a stiff back and hip misalignment, knocking on your door like uninvited guests.

And athletes aren't exempt. Certain sports involve being dominant on one side, which creates imbalances. Before long, you start hearing:

"I used to play soccer…"

"I used to play tennis…"

"I used to play golf…"

Why did they stop? Because the stress added up, and eventually, their kinetic chain called it quits.

This gradual dysfunction leads to the classic scenario: you bend over one day to pick up something tiny, like a sock or a peanut, and maybe you sneeze, "Achoo!" and your back goes out. Or your hip starts hurting "for no reason." But there *was* a reason: misalignment.

Understanding the kinetic chain is essential for staying functional.

About that phrase, "I used to…"

It breaks my heart how many people lose their ability to be active, not because of injuries or aging, but because of a trust in an industry that does not have the answers. I know I sound like a broken record about that outdated thinking. It's just that I see people with joint pain every day, knees bowed in or out, young athletes relying on painkillers, people using canes and walkers long before they should, and the constant limping. Seeing this only makes me more determined to challenge the system, change the conversation, and give people a real path to move without pain instead of managing it for the rest of their lives.

Now it's time for a little history lesson with humor.

Arthritis has been found in human remains dating back to 4000 BC. That means people have been sitting around rubbing their knees since the dawn of civilization.

Then, in the 1890s, the term "osteoarthritis" was introduced. And guess what? Over a century later, we're still telling people the same three things:

- Lose weight.
- Strengthen your leg muscles.
- Keep moving.

If we're still getting the same advice as Egyptian pharaohs... maybe it's time to rethink things.[1]

If you have tightness, soreness, stiffness, or tenderness anywhere and it lasts longer than thirty days, that's your kinetic chain trying to have a heart-to-heart with you. Don't ignore it. It will come back stronger (and not in a good way).

By now, you've likely experienced a few of the warning signs (stiffness, limping, recurring pain) telling you that your kinetic chain is out of balance. I know them well. And after ten years of searching, testing, and living this reality, I developed an extraordinary solution: **The Knee Pain Recipe**.

Welcome. It's time to reclaim your freedom.

---

[1] Jennifer Nalewicki, "3500-Year-Old Burial of Nubian Woman Reveals One of the World's Earliest Known Cases of Rheumatoid Arthritis," *Live Science*, February 9, 2024, https://www.livescience.com/archaeology/ancient-egyptians/3500-year-old-burial-of-nubian-woman-reveals-1-of-worlds-earliest-known-cases-of-rheumatoid-arthritis.

6

THE RECIPE THAT STOPPED 20 YEARS OF KNEE PAIN

You might be wondering, *What exactly is The Knee Pain Recipe?*

Well, think of it like the world's most important cookbook, but instead of ending with a delicious meal, you end with knees you will learn to love again. It is a holistic healing approach designed to reduce your knee pain using natural, strategic ingredients.

Why do I call it a recipe?

Because it took me ten years, yes, a whole decade, to blend all these remedies into one perfect sequence that actually works. This recipe has **six steps** that must be followed in order. Skip a step, and you won't get the magical "Oh my goodness, is this what relief feels like?" outcome your knees deserve.

The ingredients in this recipe are all holistic and include things like water, exfoliation, massage, stretching, kinetic-chain correction, and stability and strengthening exercises.

You might be thinking, Can I actually do this myself?

YES, you absolutely can! This method is about empowerment, taking back control of your knee health. We love doctors, but let's be honest:

you don't need an office visit every time your knees act up. This, you can handle.

Let's break it down:

Step One: Heal from the Inside Out
If your pain has been hanging around for six months… a year… five years… or even a decade, that means inflammation has moved in, set up furniture, and started getting mail.
Our first step is to evict it kindly but firmly.

Step Two: Detox and Flow The Lymphatic System
Wake up your body's natural cleanup crew and let healing fluids move freely. This is your internal cleanup crew. When you help your lymphatic system do its job, your body can finally start healing like it's supposed to.

Step Three: Ankle Mobility Secrets
In other words, you are helping your entire body work together harmoniously again.
And yes, your Knee Pain Reduction Strap plays the starring role here. (Think of it as the "main seasoning" in this recipe.)

Step Four: Creating Mobility Magic
This is where we bring back full-body movement and range of motion.
Translation: It's time to start moving like a teenager but without the drama.

Stage Five: Building Foundational Stability
Now that the body is aligned, it's time to reinforce it. A strong, stable foundation means long-lasting results.

Step Six: Strength & Resilience
The finishing touch: build real strength and endurance so pain stays gone and performance thrives.
Corrective strengthening exercises take you from pain to performance.

Yeah!!

I'm excited. I hope you are.

Experience the renewed energy and confidence of living pain-free by following these six essential steps.

SCAN THE QR CODE:

The aim of The Knee Pain Recipe is to keep your knees healthy and pain-free. After ten years of combining these ingredients, I found a way to relieve my knee pain. To achieve lasting relief, we must prepare the foundation for your healing process.

It's just like making a pie. To get the best results, you must follow the recipe in order:

1. Make the crust.
2. Prepare the filling.
3. Roll and fit the bottom crust.
4. Add filling.
5. Top the crust.
6. Finish.
7. Bake.

For ten years, it was trial and error. Then, in 2014, I broke the code on healing my knees.

I had to take it step by step to prepare my knees and body for exercise. This is the essence of my message: you need to build a strong foundation.

That year, I successfully completed what I like to call my victory lap: a 40-mile walk over two days. I walked a marathon on the first day and finished the rest on the second day. During this event, I tested my knee pain remedy to see if it worked.

And guess what? That day marked my claim to freedom: freedom from the orthopedic industry, freedom from ever needing a total knee replacement, and freedom to manage my own maintenance program. It took me decades to figure it all out, but the good news is that I can now share this information with you so you won't have to go through the same thing.

We'll take this step by step so you understand what's happening in your body. My goal is for you to feel empowered to regain control over your knees.

So, let's dive in.

7

HEALING FROM THE INSIDE OUT

STEP ONE

Knee Note: The Knee Pain Recipe is effective for the vast majority of people because it addresses what is most often ignored: alignment, circulation, and lymphatic flow. That said, certain medications, such as statins, Coumadin, and some blood pressure drugs, can actually contribute to ongoing joint pain. Scar tissue from past surgeries may block lymphatic drainage, and conditions like neuropathy, sciatica, or rheumatoid arthritis can complicate the healing process. In these cases, the Recipe can still reduce inflammation and swelling, but natural healing has limits when medications or past surgeries continue to interfere with the body's ability to recover. Even if you fall into these categories, many people still experience relief.

Healing from the inside means that the recipe starts with reducing inflammation before anything else. There are 4 healing stages to step 1.

Healing Stage 1 is where we slow things down, reduce the inflammation, and give your knee the relief it has been asking for.

Inflammation was a constant challenge during my years of pain. This is a term many of you have likely heard repeatedly.

The two main types of inflammation are acute and chronic.

- Acute inflammation is a short-term response to a sudden injury or infection and helps the body heal.
- Chronic inflammation is a long-term, ongoing immune response that can cause damage to the body over months or years and is linked to many diseases.

Chronic inflammation can lead to tissue damage, nutritional deficiencies, and accelerated aging of the joints. This is particularly relevant for people suffering from knee problems. In addition to chronic knee pain, you are also experiencing chronic inflammation, which complicates the process of alleviating the pain.

If the knee remains unhealed, inflammation will persist daily. The longer this inflammation persists, the more damage it causes to the tissues, including ligaments and cartilage. Eventually, this can lead to osteoarthritis and, in some cases, the need for a knee replacement. My goal is to teach you how to stop this chronic inflammation in your knee.

It's important to recognize that inflammation does have its benefits. It is the body's natural response to infection, helps with injuries, and assists in removing debris and damaged cells. Initially, inflammation can be beneficial, but it becomes problematic when it persists for months or even years.

How do we break the cycle of inflammation and swelling? The first step is through exfoliation. You may have heard of exfoliation in the context of skincare, where it promotes clear and soft skin. However, it also stimulates the lymphatic system. You will learn more about the lymphatic system in Step Two.

Okay, let's break this down clearly.

To begin your healing journey, I want to share how to gently break the cycle of recurring pain, inflammation, and swelling. Our first step is simple but powerful: clearing out the debris and toxicity that linger within the body. One of the most nurturing ways to do this is through hydrotherapy.

What Is Hydrotherapy?

It's a cleansing practice that detoxifies your body, awakens your lymphatic system, and prepares your spirit for healing. My method uses hot and cold showers or warm and cool showers—nothing complicated, just the elements working in your favor. However, before you begin, it's essential to create a peaceful, spiritual environment that welcomes healing.

Follow these four healing stages in order.

Healing Stage One: Create Your Sacred Space

(Scan the QR code and receive all 6 steps of the recipe in one program; see page 51)

Set aside about an hour for yourself. This is *your* time. Walk into the bathroom as if you're preparing for a normal shower, but today, we're transforming it into a healing space.

Bring a candle. Choose soothing music. Let your family know you need uninterrupted space for healing. When you step inside, light the candle and, if you wish, place a few fresh flowers nearby. These small touches signal to your mind and body that this is special.

As you settle in, take a slow breath and repeat a gentle mantra, such as:

"I love my knees."

or

"My body is ready to heal."

Let these words soften you from the inside out.

Healing Stage Two: Exfoliation and Awakening the Lymphatic System

Take your exfoliation glove. Sit comfortably, either on the toilet or by placing your foot on the edge of the tub. Beginning at your ankle, rub in circular motions.

If your ankles or lower legs are swollen, linger there. No rush. No counting. Just presence.

You're now waking up your lymphatic system, encouraging trapped fluid and inflammation to move so healing can begin. Continue slowly up your leg for twelve to fifteen minutes.

Breathe. Repeat your mantra. Let your spirit rest as your hands work.

Pay extra attention to the area behind the knee. This area houses several lymph nodes and tends to get congested when you've been living with chronic knee pain.

Continue exfoliating all the way to your groin. There are many lymph nodes here, too, supporting your body's natural detox process.

When you finish one leg, move lovingly to the other.

After both legs are complete, exfoliate your entire body, your arms, chest, back, belly, and even your face.

By doing this, you invite your whole body into healing.

Healing Stage Three: The Hydrotherapy Ritual

Now step into the shower.

Start with warm water. Rub your skin gently with your hands to remove dead skin cells, the same cells that were blocking your pores and slowing healing. Your skin will begin to feel alive again.

Keep repeating your mantra.

Once you feel relaxed, turn the water slightly hotter (but still comfortable). Stay in the heat for one minute.

Then, reach down and turn the water to cold.

When that cold water hits you, yes, it's shocking. But that shock summons your body's healing army. Your white blood cells rush forward, scanning your body for inflammation in your knees, shoulders, hips, and back.

Stay in the cold for thirty seconds.

Turn the water back to hot for thirty seconds.

Switch to cold for another thirty seconds.

Repeat this hot-cold cycle five times.

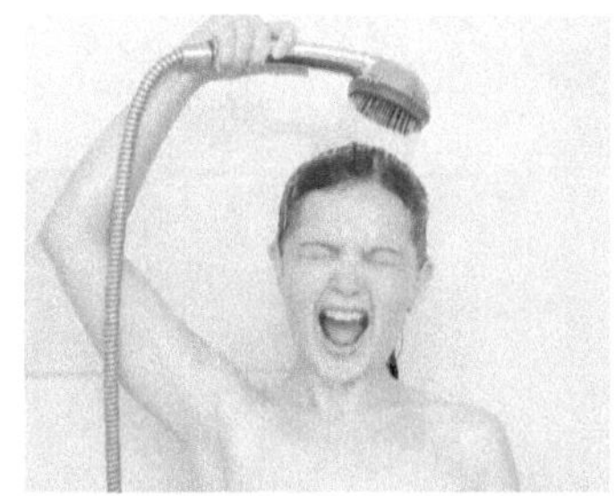

With each switch, you're flushing toxins, awakening circulation, and stimulating your lymphatic system. You're telling your body *it's time to heal.*

Healing Stage Four: Reconnection

When you finish, step out of the shower and gently dry yourself. Sit quietly on the toilet.

This is the moment when your body finally speaks.

You may feel the urge to drink water.

You may feel called to lie down.

You may feel emotion rising.

You may feel nothing but calm.

Whatever you feel, listen.

For a long time, pain has kept your mind and body disconnected, but this ritual brings them back together. Your body will guide you now. Honor its requests.

From this one session, you will notice a reduction in your knee pain. You've just experienced a simple, magical healing ritual that requires nothing more than a glove, water, and your willing participation.

You've given yourself permission to heal.

You've opened the door to a new relationship with your body.

Now you are ready to learn how to begin and stay pain-free.

8

DETOX AND FLOW: THE LYMPHATIC SYSTEM
STEP TWO

S welling is frustrating because it feels like it should be temporary. You R.I.C.E., yet it keeps coming back or never fully goes away. Prolonged pain or injury can cause the lymphatic system to become congested, trapping fluid in the joint. That's why the first step in reducing swelling is to decongest the lymphatic system.

The lymphatic system is one of the body's most sacred cleansing pathways. Think of it as your internal housekeeping crew: quiet, dedicated, and always working behind the scenes to sweep away debris and keep your body in balance.

When you're sick and those little nodes under your chin swell up, that's your lymphatic system raising its hand, saying, "I'm working overtime here!" These nodes act as tiny filters, catching what doesn't belong and helping you stay well. When this system flows freely, you feel lighter, clearer, and healthier. When it slows down, you feel... well, not your best.

My first real introduction to this powerful system came unexpectedly, during a pedicure. Yes, a pedicure! The pedicurist performed lymphatic drainage on my knees, and let me tell you, it was *not* the soothing spa moment you see in commercials. My knees were so inflamed and swollen that every touch felt intense. But that moment opened the door to the healing path I walk today. Without that experience, I may never have discovered how to eliminate my own pain, and I certainly wouldn't be here sharing this blessing with you.

In the last chapter, we talked about hydrotherapy and exfoliation. The lymphatic system works hand in hand with those practices. After your hot-and-cold shower cycles, you'll step out, sit on the commode or tub edge (whichever feels like your throne of healing), and begin your lymphatic drainage. This is the perfect time because your system is already awakened, warm, activated, and ready to release what no longer serves you.

Yes, there are professional lymphatic massage therapists who do incredible work, but I'm going to teach you how to do it yourself, Renee's way. Simple. Sacred. Effective. (See page 51 for the QR code.)

Here's something important to remember: the lymphatic system has no pump of its own, no built-in engine. You are the pump. Your hands, breath, and intention help move the lymph, especially when swelling and inflammation have made it sluggish and toxic. I'm going to show you how to reduce swelling in your knees and your ankles.

You will be amazed at how quickly you can reduce the swelling. My method is simple, gentle, and astonishingly effective. Once you feel it working, you'll look at your knees like, *Wait… that's it? That's all it took?!* Yes. That's all it took.

So, let's begin.

Imagine you've just finished your five cycles of hot and cold water. You step out of the shower, warm, refreshed, and ready.

Instead of sitting down immediately, you'll begin your lymphatic drainage.

We always start at the ankles. Always. The journey upward starts from the foundation.

What we're about to do is a special kind of massage. This is a healing practice with intention, intuition, and a sprinkle of my magical style.

To make it even easier, I've included a simple how-to video. Scan the QR code on page 51 so you can follow along step by step.

Lymphatic drainage is essential for anyone who wants to heal their body or maintain vibrant health. Ideally, everyone should get a professional lymphatic drainage massage at least twice a year. A trained therapist can detect sluggish spots throughout your body, yes, even beyond the legs. Areas you might not even realize are congested.

Most lymphatic massage therapists start at the neck and work downward, and that's a beautiful method. But when I tried to teach people the professional way, it just didn't land. Folks were looking at me like, *My knee hurts, not my neck.* So, I switched things up and started from the bottom (ankles, calves, shins), and the results were incredible. I felt a tingling in my leg, my knee pain eased, and I knew I was onto something. Sometimes, you just have to flip the script.

Remember, your lymphatic system is responsible for ushering toxins, waste, and bacteria out of your body. And trust me, you want that stuff gone. When lymph fluid gets stuck, your entire system suffers.

Now let's talk about something we *all* know too well...

Why Your Knees Hurt When It Rains

Back in the day, our grandparents didn't need a weather app. They'd just stand up, wince, and say, *"Rain's coming."* And somehow... They were always right.

If your knees start complaining the minute the clouds roll in, you are not alone, and no, you are not turning into a human barometer for no reason.

When it rains, barometric pressure drops. For someone with osteoarthritis, this change can cause the knee to swell even more. That swelling traps lymphatic fluid in the lymph nodes around the knee. When those nodes fill up, they start pressing on your nerve endings. That pressure is what causes the deep, throbbing ache, not just in your knees, but sometimes in your shoulders, hips, and even your back. Your body isn't being dramatic; it's reacting to a weather shift.

I'll never forget the day I discovered what I now call my *"rain massage."* I was sitting on my sofa, my knees hurting so badly I was on the verge of tears. Desperate, I instinctively started massaging the area behind my knee. I had no idea what I was doing; I wasn't being thera-peutic, I was being desperate.

When I finished, the pain was gone. Just… gone.

That moment stopped me in my tracks. I later learned that the area behind the knee houses lymph nodes. When the knee swells, fluid can't pass through properly. The lymph nodes fill up with nowhere to drain, and your nerves pay the price. Once the pressure is released, relief follows.

I can assume you never thought your knees would become the weather reporter.

On another occasion, while sitting at my table during another episode of pain, I invented what I call the "inner and outer massage." I massaged the inside of my knee, then used my hand to gently push excess fluid up to my lymph nodes. The pain melted away. I did the same thing to the outside of my knee, and boom, relief again. This is an excellent technique for people with meniscus tears.

Every technique I share with you was born out of real pain, real trial and error, and real healing.

And now they're here for *you*.

Pain from Sitting, Driving, or Getting Out of Bed

Here's a simple technique I created for those who sit at a desk, whether they're working hard or scrolling TikTok. I won't judge!

While sitting, place your hands under your knees and gently perform lymph drainage. Then tap your feet on the floor, yes, just like you're listening to music, especially jazz. This stimulates your lymphatic system, which doesn't have its own pump.

When you stand afterward, you'll notice something amazing: no stiffness. This one trick can save you from years of unnecessary pain.

Healing Isn't Complicated

So many people feel discouraged, believing that pain is just their new normal. But healing is possible.

If you commit to understanding and practicing my systems, you will be amazed at how quickly swelling in your ankles and knees disappears right before your eyes.

This book exists to help you reclaim your knee health. Yes, I still recommend receiving a full lymphatic drainage massage every six months. A professional can tell you things about your body you may never notice on your own.

The real key to healing?

Stay proactive. Stay consistent. Stay hopeful.

When people first begin my program, consistency is crucial. Some people have reduced their pain by 50 percent in a matter of days once the inflammation has been reduced. You will see the transformation in the first thirty to forty-five days: less stiffness and swelling, more movement, and hope.

As for me?

I no longer need to perform The Knee Pain Recipe. However, I do teach The Moten Method: two classes per day, four days a week, to women all over the world. My knees have healed, and so have those of the women in my classes. As of 2026, I've taught over 1,660 online classes exclusively for women with hip, back, shoulder, and, of course, knee pain.

My Reality Today

Today, in 2026, I live knee-pain-free.

Yes, I still have osteoarthritis in both knees and hips.

I occasionally practice the lymphatic routine simply as maintenance, like watering a plant.

I'm not here to teach you how to *manage* pain.

I'm here to teach you how to **eliminate** it.

If you commit just five hours a week to my system, you can reduce knee, hip, and back pain and start reclaiming your life.

Your Healing Journey

I recommend pairing lymph drainage with:

- Hot and cold showers.
- Exfoliation.
- Gentle lymphatic massage.

This combination is powerful, and yes, you can do it daily.

The more you do it, the quicker you break the pain cycle.

Keep reading. Keep learning. Keep healing.

I'm with you every step of the way on this journey.

9

HEALING BEGINS AT THE ANKLE

STEP THREE

Your body is a brilliant problem-solver, sometimes too brilliant. It constantly compensates for old injuries, weaknesses, or imbalances by creating a "custom" movement pattern (a.k.a. your gait). The problem? These patterns often place unnatural stress on joints and tissues far from where the issue began. So, while you're blaming your knee, your walking gait might be the real troublemaker.

This book will show you exactly how your gait exposes the hidden causes of your pain so you can finally fix the root issue, not chase symptoms.

But pay attention: these steps must be done in order to get real, lasting results.

First, we detox the system, reduce inflammation, and minimize swelling. You cannot heal in an inflammatory swamp. Clearing swelling and supporting your lymphatic system while rebalancing the kinetic chain is non-negotiable.

Again, these steps must occur together. Why? Because the way you walk right now is likely making everything worse. If you're limping (or even "micro-limping," and you know who you are), you're adding inflammation and extra stress to your back, knees, and hips. Skip this part, and you'll get partial relief at best.

And please, don't overlook getting my Knee Pain Reduction Strap System® and a proper gait analysis.[1] One supports your healing in real time, and the other reveals exactly why you're in pain in the first place. Your knees will thank you. Your back will thank you.

This is where the knee pain reduction strap, mentioned earlier, becomes essential. You will need this tool to help rebalance the kinetic chain, which will ultimately stop the limping and prevent further inflammation and swelling.

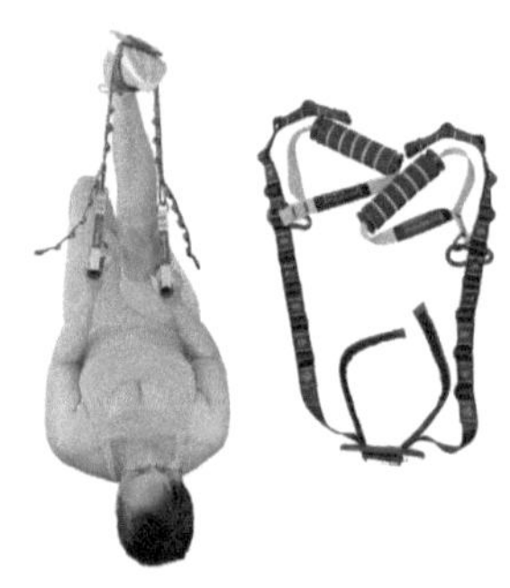

Visualize a single, versatile tool engineered to stretch, strengthen, and stabilize your body's entire kinetic chain.

SCAN THE QR CODE:

All joint healing starts at the ankle. According to the Harvard Newsletter, "Healthy ankles: Your mobility depends on them.[2] The third step in The Knee Pain Recipe is to re-establish full range of motion in the ankles, calves, shins, and feet. These few stretches and exercises are crucial to bringing the body back into balance.

---

1. Health Publishing, "Healthy Ankles: Your Mobility Depends on Them," *Harvard Health Publishing*,https://www.health.harvard.edu/pain/healthy-ankles-your-mobility-depends-on-them.

2. Harvard Health Publishing, "Healthy Ankles: Your Mobility Depends on Them," *Harvard Health Publishing*, June 18, 2015, https://www.health.harvard.edu/pain/healthy-ankles-your-mobility-depends-on-them.

- Tennis ball rolling
- Toe Raises
- Ankle circles
- Calf raises
- Windshield wipers

A Gift for You: "Prioritizing ankle health can help to prevent knee surgery and restore our independence."

SCAN THE QR CODE:

Why Is This Step So Important?

We have become a nation of sitters. Sitting for long periods at school, at the office, at home, or while driving causes the muscles in front of the hip to shorten and weaken and the muscles in the back to become overstretched. That is a combination that can cause an injury.

Have you ever stood up from a seated position and found it necessary to lean backward in order to stretch your back? You are stretching your hip flexor muscles. One of the muscles, the psoas, is attached to the front of the hip and to the lumbar spine at the L4 and L5 regions.

Because of prolonged sitting and a lack of daily stretching, walking or jogging with shortened or overstretched muscles can cause an uneven gait. Your feet may flare out like a duck's, your hips may lack movement, and your arms may rest by your sides instead of swinging.

Your gait is crucial because it reflects whether your body mechanics are functioning correctly. It can reveal imbalances in your movement.

What Is Involved with a Walking Gait Analysis?

You will need another person, if possible. I suggest walking away from the camera at least fifteen steps, then walking back toward the camera.

These fifteen steps will tell a lot about why you are still in pain. To receive a free gait analysis report, send your video to Reneemoten@ healmyknees.com.

The gait analysis can be your first defense against ever developing knee, hip, and back pain.

> **Knee Note:** *I walked incorrectly for years, and then one day, I performed a squat, and my right knee started hurting. If anyone had performed a gait analysis in 1993, I would not be writing this book. That's how important a gait analysis can be. Life-changing.*

Treadmill walkers and runners, listen closely: do both feet strike the treadmill evenly? If one foot hits the platform harder than the other, it indicates an imbalance that you must address before starting an exercise routine.

By investing your time in an analysis, you can gain valuable feedback to improve balance and alignment. Let's ensure you are well-prepared for successful walks, jogging sessions, and exercise programs. Don't postpone getting that gait analysis.

When discussing footwear, people ask me, "Renee, what kind of shoes should I buy?" This is especially true for those with knee problems. They want to know which shoes will alleviate their discomfort. My response is usually, "You shouldn't buy any new shoes right now."

They often look confused and ask why. I explain that they are not walking correctly. Until they undergo a gait analysis and rebalance their muscles, purchasing new shoes won't help. Feet can't effectively absorb impact if they are not hitting the ground properly.

First, we'll focus on getting your body into alignment; then we can find the right shoes that will truly support you.

I also noticed that most of the attendees in my classes were women, which made me curious about why so many women experience knee problems.

Research from the NIH supports this observation, highlighting that women are more likely than men to experience osteoarthritis and that the severity of knee arthritis tends to be greater in women.[3]

The statistics are astonishing: out of 325 million people with osteoarthritis (OA), 60 percent are women.[4]

I wondered what sets women apart from men in this regard. Then it struck me: the issue often lies in our footwear.

Women love a good fashion moment, and let's be honest, we will squeeze, pinch, cram, and contort our feet into a shoe if it completes the outfit. Comfort? Support? Arch stability? I look good. I will deal with that later. Unfortunately, "later" usually shows up as corns, calluses, bunions, and a whole lot of unnecessary suffering. And yes, women lead the scoreboard in all three.

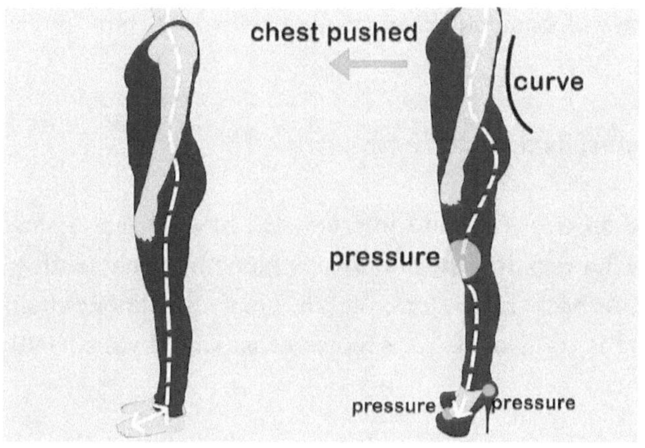

I've seen more bunions than I can count. Bunions caused by high heels, bunions caused by tight shoes, and bunions caused by "the shoes were on sale, so I had to get them." High heels place all your weight onto

---

3. Sharon L. Hame and Reginald A. Alexander, "Knee Osteoarthritis in Women," *Current Reviews in Musculoskeletal Medicine* 6, no. 2 (June 2013): 182,https://pmc.ncbi.nlm.nih.gov/articles/PMC3702776/.

4. World Health Organization, "Osteoarthritis," World Health Organization, July 14, 2023, https://www.who.int/news-room/fact-sheets/detail/osteoarthritis.

the front of your foot, especially the balls of your feet, and your poor big toe joint starts expanding like it's trying to escape the situation entirely. That's how that famous (or infamous) bump forms.

It's honestly shocking how many bunions I see on women's feet. And don't get me started on the high heels, backless shoes, and "cute but no arch support whatsoever" styles we love so much. And when we finally sit in a pedicure chair? We don't ask why we have calluses. Nope. We just say, "Shave them off. I am wearing sandals, and I need my feet to look good."

But that mindset is exactly what leads to knee pain later on.

Here's the truth: bunions, calluses, and corns are not random—they're *messages*. Your body is waving a red flag, saying, *Hey! Something's wrong with the way you walk!* And until we choose footwear that actually supports us, shoes with a real back, real structure, and real arch support, we're going to keep dealing with foot, hip, and even back problems.

Knee note: *Bunions can be hereditary*

In more than two thousand interviews, I haven't met a single person with only knee pain. There's always something happening with the feet, hips, or back, right along with it. That's the kinetic chain at work; everything is connected. Your footwear is part of your health, not just your outfit.

Now, if you are going to rock your heels (because, let's be honest, we're not giving them up), you MUST learn how to stretch properly before you wear them, while you're wearing them, and after you take them off. My Knee Pain Reduction Strap is one of the best tools you can use to stretch your feet, protect your knees and hips, and keep you looking fabulous without paying the price later.

And let me say this loud and clear: stretching isn't optional; it's a lifestyle. If you want to keep your joints healthy, improve your gait, and stay pain-free as long as possible, the Knee Pain Reduction Strap should be at the very top of your toolkit.

Because, yes, you can be stylish and pain-free. You just need to stop letting your shoes call the shots.

10

CREATING MOBILITY MAGIC

STEP FOUR

Can a Holistic System Really Give You Back Your Freedom? **Yes, it can.**

The Moten Method ushers in a new era of pain reduction.

This method is a step-by-step transformation exercise system that relieves knee pain, restores movement, and slows the damaging progression of osteoarthritis, all without drugs, injections, or surgery.

In 2014, I created *The Knee Pain Recipe* not because I had all the answers, but because I was determined to protect my newly discovered pain-free life. After years of knee drama, I wasn't about to hand my knees back to chaos. Something was clearly working, but I didn't yet know which stretches and exercises were my knees' best friends… and which ones were secretly plotting against me.

Then the world shut down. When COVID arrived, I was suddenly forced online with a small group of brave, trusting clients who were willing to experiment with me.

What felt like a major obstacle, COVID turned into a gift. Those unexpected years became my real-life laboratory.

Together, we tested exercises, immediately fired the ones that caused flare-ups, and kept only what truly worked. Knees, by the way, are wonderfully honest. They don't whisper their opinions. They send a loud, swollen memo the moment you make a bad decision.

By 2021, I had cracked the code. I learned how to teach ten different types of knee-safe routines that build strength *without* triggering inflammation. These routines included cardio, balance, chair work, floor work, coordination, tubing, medicine ball training, high- and low-intensity routines, programs for total knee replacement and bone-on-bone knees, and lymphatic drainage. Yes, the knees were busy, but not angry.

After refining and perfecting these routines over the next three years (and listening closely to every knee complaint), the system was finally ready to step out into the world.

That's when **The Moten Method** was born.

It brings together *The Knee Pain Recipe*, the Knee Pain Reduction Strap, and a complete, thoughtful system designed to help people move with confidence again, without fear, flare-ups, or regret.

This method was created from experience, persistence, and love. Love for the health and wellness industry, love for my clients, and love for my business, Heal My Knees.

Because knees deserve patience, kindness, and yes, a little laughter along the way.

The Moten Method empowers you to prevent future setbacks, rebuild resilience, and reclaim an active, fulfilling life… without your knees filing formal complaints.

Why The Moten Method Works

I named this program after myself because I believe it's one of the most effective foundational programs in the world. With over twenty-seven years of experience in fitness and health and nearly twenty-four years focused on knee issues, I've seen firsthand what works and what doesn't. The structure of The Moten Method is sound, proven, and safe. I'm proud to attach my name to it because it delivers results.

The Moten Method targets the true sources of knee pain:

- Misalignment of the kinetic chain
- Limping shoe patterns
- Restricted ankle mobility
- Dysfunctional upper body mechanics

This program doesn't just manage discomfort; it slows deterioration before the knee deformity sets in. It restores proper body mechanics and stabilizes your body by using corrective exercises.

Knee Note: This book is not about giving you another list of exercises to stabilize or strengthen your leg muscles. We all have been there and done that. This is about giving you the opportunity to take control of your health and wellness.
*The collection of stretches and stabilizing exercises you will find here is part of a much bigger system. I call it your **maintenance library**, designed to support you once you are out of pain. Here is an OCR code for over 80 stretches and stabilizing exercises.*

Experience a collection of 80 proven exercises and stretches, expertly designed for maximum efficiency, effectiveness, and safety.

SCAN THE QR CODE:

The Role of the Knee Pain Reduction Strap

A cornerstone of The Moten Method is my patented Knee Pain Reduction Strap. This isn't a brace; it's a revolutionary tool that:

- Strengthens and stretches in both inversion and eversion of the ankle.
- Helps prevent ankle rolling, which often leads to the end of careers for athletes.
- Provides 11 stretches for full ankle and leg range of motion.
- Fits easily in your car, gym bag, or suitcase.

The strap helps improve ankle stability, which is critical because ankle injuries often lead to knee pain, as I learned firsthand. Using this strap consistently can reduce tension on your knees, improve alignment, and support long-term joint health.

Understanding Your Knee Issues

Osteoarthritis (OA) is a degenerative joint disease where the protective cartilage that cushions the ends of bones gradually breaks down. In advanced stages, this can cause the bones to rub together, leading to inflammation, pain, stiffness, and reduced mobility. Maintaining proper alignment and mechanics is essential for managing the condition and supporting joint health throughout life.

The four stages of osteoarthritis, often classified using the Kellgren-Lawrence grading system, are:

- **Stage One (Minor):** Characterized by minor wear and tear and very small bone spurs (osteophytes), usually with little to no pain or symptoms.
- **Stage Two (Mild):** More noticeable bone spurs are visible on X-rays. Sufferers may experience mild stiffness after prolonged inactivity or pain after activity, but the cartilage gap is typically still healthy.
- **Stage Three (Moderate):** Cartilage begins to significantly erode, narrowing the space between bones. The joint becomes inflamed, causing more frequent pain and stiffness during daily activities.
- **Stage Four (Severe):** This is the end stage, where cartilage is almost completely gone, leading to bone-on-bone contact. Pain

is often constant and severe, and joint deformity may occur, making daily activities difficult.

Meniscus Tears: The meniscus is a thick, rubbery piece of cartilage that sits inside the knee joint. You have two of them in each knee, one on the inside and one on the outside. Their job is to act like shock absorbers, cushioning the bones and helping the knee stay stable during walking, bending, and twisting.

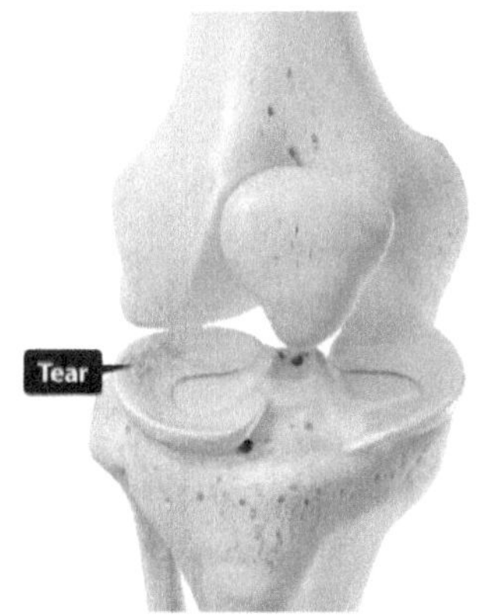

Knee Note: The meniscus doesn't usually "tear" because it's weak. It gets damaged when the knee is forced to move improperly, often because the body is compensating for problems elsewhere in the kinetic chain. Limping, poor foot mechanics, stiff ankles, or hip imbalance can overload the meniscus step after step until it finally gives way.

Meniscus tears come in various shapes and sizes, and they often lead to secondary issues, like a Baker's cyst, which forms as inflammatory fluid collects at the back of the knee. While surgery can sometimes remove damaged tissue, addressing any underlying biomechanical imbalances is the key to long-term joint stability.

The common classifications for meniscus tears based on their appearance or pattern include:

- **Radial Tear:** This tear starts at the inner edge of the meniscus and extends outward, perpendicular to the main fibers. They are often in the "white zone" (an area with reduced blood flow) and typically require surgical intervention.
- **Longitudinal Tear:** These run lengthwise along the meniscus, parallel to its circumference. Depending on their location in the vascular "red zone," they may have the

potential to heal on their own or with repair. A complete longitudinal tear can displace, forming a **bucket-handle tear**.

- **Horizontal Tear:** A tear that splits the meniscus into upper and lower portions, parallel to the shin bone (tibia). These can sometimes be treated non-surgically, particularly if they are degenerative.
- **Flap Tear:** A tear where a piece of the meniscus becomes detached but remains tethered, creating a flap that can cause catching or locking sensations in the knee. This tear usually needs surgery.
- **Complex/Degenerative Tear:** These involve a combination of two or more tear patterns (e.g., radial, horizontal, and flap) and often result from age-related wear and tear.

Treatment options depend heavily on the type, size, and location of the tear, as well as the patient's age and activity level.

What type of meniscus tear do you have? Do not leave it up to the doctor to make your decision about surgery. Get yourself educated and take an active role in your surgery and healing.

Patellofemoral Syndrome (PFS)

Patellofemoral syndrome is irritation and breakdown that occurs under the kneecap, where the patella is supposed to glide smoothly over the thigh bone. When everything is working properly, the kneecap tracks effortlessly with each step, squat, or bend of the knee. But when the kinetic chain is out of alignment, that smooth tracking disappears.

Bone-on-Bone

"Bone-on-bone" is one of the most frightening phrases a person can hear about their knees, and it's also one of the most misunderstood.

In most cases, true bone-on-bone contact is not actually happening.

As long as the meniscus is intact, the bones of the knee are separated. The meniscus acts as a spacer and shock absorber, keeping the femur and tibia from directly grinding against each other, even when X-rays are labeled "severe arthritis."

What imaging often shows is **loss of joint space**, cartilage thinning, or changes in bone shape. That does not automatically mean bone is slamming into bone with every step. Yet the language alone convinces people they are fragile, broken, and out of options.

And that fear changes how they move.

> **Knee Note:** *Need surgery? There are cases where knee pain has been present for so long that the cartilage has significantly deteriorated, leading to joint deformity or near-total cartilage loss. In situations like these, surgery may become unavoidable. When that happens,* **The Moten Method** *becomes essential. This method is designed to prepare the body for surgery in a way no other program does.*

All of these conditions can be treated without drugs, shots, or surgery. The **Knee Pain Recipe** teaches you how to reduce swelling, restore mobility, and prevent further damage before attempting any strengthening exercises. Healing always comes first.

Lessons from the Field

Over more than twenty years, I've worked with:

- People with meniscus tears, patellofemoral syndrome, OA, and post-surgery knees.
- Clients with hip, back, and shoulder problems caused by long-term misalignment.
- Physical therapists, instructors, trainers, and even doctors seeking solutions they couldn't find elsewhere.

I've observed hundreds of classes and seen how common exercises, such as lunges, squats, and jumping jacks, are often taught incorrectly, causing more pain than progress. My method emphasizes safe, corrective movement, proper form, and mindful alignment.

Remember: Ankle injuries can lead to knee pain, knee pain can lead to hip pain, and poor mechanics can affect your entire body. By following The Moten Method, you are not just managing symptoms; you are reclaiming your life.

Understanding the Knee Joint

Understanding your knee condition often means looking at the bigger picture of joint health and biology. For many female athletes, particularly in high-impact sports like basketball and volleyball, the frequency of ACL tears is higher than in men. A key factor contributing to this disparity is related to hormones, specifically estrogen.

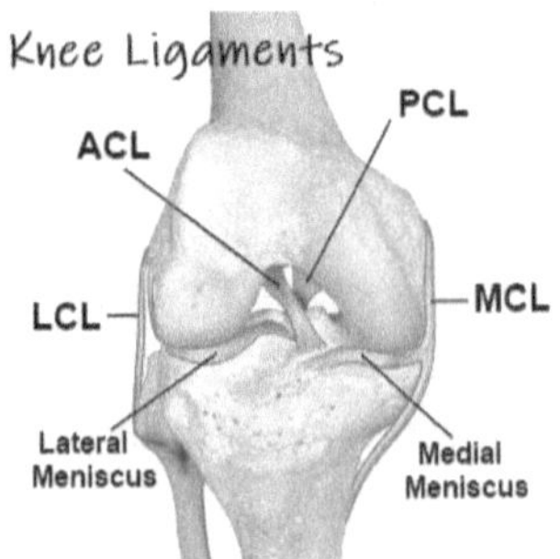

The Mechanism of Estrogen's Effect

Estrogen can influence the integrity of the anterior cruciate ligament (ACL):

- **Decreased Ligament Stiffness and Strength:** When estrogen levels are high (such as during certain phases of the menstrual cycle), the hormone may cause the ligament tissue to become less stiff and weaker.
- **Reduced Load Tolerance:** A weaker ligament is less able to withstand the normal biomechanical loads and stresses encountered during physical activity, increasing the risk of a non-contact tear.

Knee Note: Ligaments are strong bands of connective tissue that connect bones to other bones within a joint. They provide stability, limit excessive movement, and help prevent joint dislocation. They do not stretch.

The knee joint is made up mostly of ligaments. This is what makes the knee one of the strongest joints in the body. Remember, ligaments connect bone to bone, which is why their strength is so vital.

However, in young girls and women, due to estrogen, there is a slight laxity in these ligaments, which can create more vulnerability because of the hormonal influence. They can try to strengthen themselves as much as possible, but they will always have a slight disadvantage due to estrogen.

Another factor is that girls have a Q-angle, which can cause significant pulling on the IT band. The Moten Method has developed a coach's manual on protecting the knee and preventing lower ACL injuries. (see chapter 12)

Next, let's discuss the **MCL** (medial collateral ligament). MCL injuries are similar to ACL (anterior cruciate ligament) tears. Both involve tears, but their locations differ: the MCL is on the medial (inner) side of the knee, while the ACL is on the front of the knee.

MCL injuries are not as common, but when they do occur, they are still tears. Once torn, they need to be addressed. In some cases, a small tear may remain manageable for an extended period. However, MCL tears often necessitate knee surgery. Why is this necessary? Because a torn MCL can lead to knee instability, increasing the risk of falls and further damage.

You may need to get it fixed, even if it's just a small tear.

Patellar tendinitis, commonly known as "jumper's knee," affects many basketball players, who engage in repetitive jumping. This can be remedied with the knee pain recipe and the strap.

It's important to understand what tendinitis means. Remember, a tendon connects muscle to bone. If there is a misalignment in the knee joint from a muscle imbalance, this will put strain on the tendon. As a result, the tendon can become inflamed, leading to tendinitis.

In the case of patellar tendinitis, you're essentially pulling too much on the tendon attached to your kneecap, known as the patella. This repeated strain can cause inflammation.

To recover, follow a three-step process. While I may sound repetitive, these steps will help reduce inflammation and get you back on track. Typically, recovery can take anywhere from three weeks to thirty days, not years. However, the orthopedic industry often allows these injuries and pains to persist for a long time, using shots and braces instead of working to realign the kinetic chain.

So, what alternatives do we have? For various types of knee injuries and problems, that's where The Moten Method comes into play as your saving grace. The Moten Method will show you how to return to the person you once were, your old self.

One important aspect I realized was that I couldn't tackle this journey on my own. I needed to build a team of professionals to help me. For instance, I found it essential to see a certified lymphatic drainage therapist. While I can teach you some lymphatic drainage techniques, it's crucial to consult a professional.

Additionally, you should consider getting regular stretching sessions (after your pain has decreased). There are many stretching studios worldwide, and they can help identify if you're tighter on one side than the other.

Another vital resource is a kinesiology chiropractor. They can help determine if you're truly in alignment or if you still need to make adjustments. It's important to recognize that we need support from others on this journey, and that's what this holistic team can provide for you.

My programs will help you engage effectively with these professionals. The Moten Method will guide you before visiting a lymphatic drainage therapist to receive specific guidelines. The same goes for stretching sessions and kinesiology chiropractic appointments. That's the essence of The Moten Method. Scan the QR code on page 51 and choose a life-changing program.

The program will provide guidelines to help you make the most of your visits to these professionals.

I personally see my team every six months to ensure I'm staying in alignment. This is crucial, especially since I have osteoarthritis in my knees and hips. If I become misaligned, I need to address it right away.

That's why it's important to have your team and to visit them every six months, not every week or month. The Moten Method will give you the tools.

Now, let's wrap up our discussion about The Moten Method, as I'm excited to move on to the next phase.

The Moten Method provides a range of tools to treat various types of injuries, along with your support team. Here are some of the tools included:

1. Full body stretch
2. Movement patterns (I'll explain this later)
3. Inner and outer massage
4. Baker's cyst reduction
5. Gait analysis
6. Toe yoga
7. Kneecap movement
8. Trigger point therapy

There are techniques that you may not have heard of before. As I mentioned at the beginning of this chapter, I wish someone had informed me about the various available alternatives.

Understand that navigating these methods is not simple or easy. Health and wellness require time, patience, and discipline. However, the outcome is incredibly empowering. You can learn to alleviate your pain through self-care and use these techniques for a lifetime.

While we certainly need medical professionals, self-management is also key. That's why The Moten Method was created: to help people like you and me get back to our true selves.

Helping people to reduce their knee pain without drugs, shots, or surgery needs to be spread around the world. Below, I would like to introduce you to **The Moten Method Certification Program.**

If you are a personal trainer, massage therapist, or physical therapist, I would appreciate your help. As I mentioned earlier, I've observed that many health, wellness, and fitness professionals work around joint pain when in the gym or on the massage table. Most massage therapists will not even touch the knee in fear of causing pain. Learning my techniques and methods can really enhance a health and wellness practitioner's confidence and overall bottom line.

This certification program will guide you through various stages of instruction and, most importantly, provide over 150 exercises suited to online and in-person sessions, all while ensuring participant safety. Many people attending these classes lack proper stretching and come in with the expectation that the instructor will guide them and keep them safe; unfortunately, that is often not the case.

My certification program lasts for six months. During this time, you will learn foundational skills that are essential before you can start teaching your desired topics. It's crucial to understand how participants' feet should properly hit a step, how they should move to the side, and where their arms and hips should be positioned to prevent injury.

This training is desperately needed in our industry. Right now, both instructors and students are at risk of injury, and it doesn't have to be this way. We simply need to approach instruction differently. If you want more information, just push on the OCR code. Let's chat.

Looking to join forces with wellness innovators and those strategic thinkers who challenge the status quo.

SCAN THE QR CODE:

11

BUILDING FOUNDATIONAL STABILITY

STEP FIVE

Your knees are some of the hardest-working and most underappreciated joints in your body. They absorb the shock of nearly every step, squat, and stair climb, all while carrying your full body weight. So when your knees hurt, it's not just inconvenient; it can instantly change how you move, how confident you feel, and how much you trust your own body.

Here's the part most people don't realize (and no one tells you): your knees don't work alone. And let me be clear: knees are terrible at multitasking for other joints.

The result? Compensation, misalignment, extra pressure, and eventually pain. Lots of it.

In this chapter, you'll learn full-body stabilization strategies that protect your knees not just for today, but for years to come. This is Step Five of The Moten Method, where we stabilize the *entire kinetic chain* to reduce unnecessary strain, prevent further cartilage damage, and help you take back control of how you move—without fear.

As I've shared before, knee problems don't discriminate. They show up at all ages. And among them, the most damaging and misunder-

85

stood diagnosis is osteoarthritis. Once cartilage begins to break down, protecting what remains becomes non-negotiable.

So let me say this clearly, and I want you to hear it twice:

If you follow my steps, you can slow down or even stop the progression of osteoarthritis.

Yes, I know. That goes directly against the traditional orthopedic message that says, "Once you have OA, surgery is just a matter of time."

The Moten Method challenges that belief. It doesn't just help you manage pain; it interrupts the very cycle that creates it in the first place.

And I'll go a step further: that traditional perspective is simply inaccurate.

I have the proof? X-rays. Plural.

I have imaging from 2000, 2004, 2011, and 2021. My knee pain diagnosis goes all the way back to the early 1990s—around 1992—when I was first told I had "joint noise." You know the sound: the snap, crackle, and pop that make you pause mid-step and wonder if your bones are breaking.

Over time, I was diagnosed with patellofemoral syndrome and later osteoarthritis in both knees. Every new report said the same thing: mild… then moderate… then hips progressively worsening. And yet here's the part that should make you curious: I still have both my knees and hips.

Think about that.

Four sets of X-rays. An MRI confirming osteoarthritis. Decades of documentation. And I am pain-free with fully functioning knees and hips.

Here's what never made sense to me.

Doctors know how to successfully treat plantar fasciitis, tendonitis, and bursitis. They understand inflammation. They understand overuse. They understand compensation.

Yet when the diagnosis becomes osteoarthritis, the conversation abruptly changes to, *"Just live with it until surgery."*

So the real question isn't whether osteoarthritis can be slowed down or even stopped.

My question is this: When athletes, active adults, and seniors come to orthopedic doctors with knee pain or injuries, why doesn't the doctor ever consider that the ankle might be the beginning of the problem? Why wasn't the entire movement chain ever part of the discussion?

There are hundreds of articles showing how limited ankle mobility can directly contribute to knee pain and breakdown. hundreds.[1] [2] [3] And yet most solutions still focus only on the knee. Using creams, drugs, braces, injections, and physical therapy protocols that never look beyond the joint itself.

What gets overlooked is the person living with chronic pain from having had an injury.

People like you and me invest valuable time, money, and hope, only to lose the mobility that knee pain took away from us. For athletes, that means watching the game instead of playing it. For others, it means quietly stepping away from the activities that once made life feel full.

That loss is personal.

Why did no one ever look at the whole picture?

---

[1] Kyle Norman, "Alleviating Knee Pain Through Ankle Mobility," *Trail Runner Magazine*, May 8, 2018, https://www.trailrunnermag.com/training/injuries-and-treatment-training/ankle-mobility-for-trail-runners/.

[2] Kade L. Paterson et al., "The Relationship between Foot and Ankle Symptoms and Risk of Developing Knee Osteoarthritis: Data from the Osteoarthritis Initiative," *Osteoarthritis and Cartilage* 25, no. 6 (June 2017): 818–25,https://pubmed.ncbi.nlm.nih.gov/27939621/.

[3] "Ankle Mobility: Understand the Link to Knee Pain," The Basketball Doctors, March 14, 2024, https://thebasketballdoctors.com/ankle-mobility-understand-the-link-to-knee-pain/.

Why didn't people from Harvard and NIH broadcast their findings about ankle mobility?

Maybe in the future I will find out.

Let's move on.

We need to understand the term "crepitus," that crunching or crackling sound you hear when climbing stairs. Many people think it's their bones grinding together, but that's not what's actually happening yet!

Your kneecap is supposed to sit in the center of the trochlear groove in your femur. Think of the groove like a fork, guiding the kneecap smoothly. When the kneecap slips slightly off center, it creates that "crunch, crunch, crunch" sound, especially when going up stairs. You won't hear it as much on flat ground because the pressure and angle aren't as intense. Crepitus is one of the signs that you are out of alignment.

Now it's time to stabilize a body that is finally ready to move without pain.

> *Knee Note: Steps one through four have prepared the body to begin this stabilization. By the fifth step, your knee pain should have decreased by 50 percent. If not, start with step one again.*

To begin this process, consider the four muscle groups in each leg:

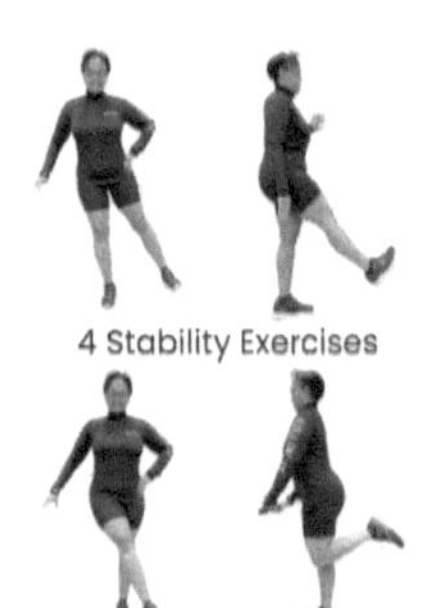

4 Stability Exercises

1. Outer thigh
2. Quadriceps (front of the leg)
3. Inner thigh
4. Hamstring (back of leg)

> *Knee Note: These exercises are not meant to be hard. The purpose is for you to listen to the muscles on the right side of your body and then*

compare the muscle strength to the left side. Both sides must feel even. (Use the QR code. See page 73.)

Focusing on these areas will improve your overall alignment. You can perform this exercise while standing or lying down, depending on your fitness level.

If you're standing, balance on your left foot and extend your right leg out to the side. Aim for 30 repetitions, and pay close attention to how your body feels. Does your leg feel weak, strong, tight, or sore?

After completing 30 reps on the right side, switch: stand on your right leg and lift your left leg 30 times. Again, notice how each side feels. Were you able to complete all 30 reps evenly? If one side is weaker, continue practicing until both sides feel balanced.

As I mentioned earlier, this book is not about giving you a list of strengthening exercises. These movements are an example of how, by balancing these four foundational muscle groups along with the full range of motion in the ankle, calf, and shin, you begin to achieve full-body stability and rebalance your kinetic chain.

This is how stability is built.

If standing is too difficult, my subscription page offers seated alternatives. You'll find three progressive levels of exercises designed for every ability.

These assessments become essential parts of your routine. They show whether you are more balanced on one side than the other, and balance is not optional. It is a requirement for knee health.

Once your body begins to feel balanced, you can move on to more advanced exercises. My programs contain a wide variety of movements that support your stability work. As you begin walking, cycling, exercising, or even lightly jogging, pay attention to how your body responds.

Why is this important?

Because as you increase your activity, about 85 percent of your knee pain should decrease as long as you've completed the earlier steps correctly. This is the turning point; when you begin to feel good, you will *want* to stay active and stay consistent.

Certain conditions indicate that you are out of alignment. Understanding these signals is crucial to your progress.

1. If your knee locks up, it means there is inflammation at the back of the knee. When this occurs, return to step one. That's how this process works.
2. If your knee suddenly gives out while walking, it often means the quadriceps tendon is inflamed and not supporting the joint properly.
3. When a tendon becomes inflamed, it sends a protective signal that "shuts off" the muscle it attaches to. This is why your knee may feel weak or unstable. To correct this, you must return to Steps One and Two, reduce inflammation, and identify the cause.
4. When taking a walk or jogging, if your calf or hamstrings tighten up or you get shin splints, go back to steps one, two, and three.
5. If you've ever wondered why your knee makes a crunching sound, the source is usually a misaligned kneecap. The iliotibial (IT) band often pulls the kneecap sideways, especially when climbing stairs or biking. Restoring alignment is essential.

Many people tell me, "Renee, I have pain in the front of my knee." That usually means their shin muscles are weak and their calves are too strong. The fix is simple: strengthen the shins.

My books, programs, and classes answer these types of questions you may have about knee pain.

Give The Moten Method **60 days** and see how much your life can change, just as it changed mine and the lives of countless others. (See page 51 for the QR code.)

12

STRENGTH & RESILIENCE

STEP SIX

When should you start strengthening?

Not while your knees are still filing complaints. Strengthening should only be introduced once pain and stiffness are gone and daily movements such as walking, stair climbing, jogging, and getting out of bed feel natural again.

Your knees did not start hurting because your legs were weak. Your knees became chronically sore because you were out of balance.

> **Knee Note:** *Prevention is always the goal. But if osteoarthritis has already developed, meaning there is cartilage damage, it's a **must** to maintain full flexibility throughout the whole body. The entire kinetic chain **must** remain aligned, and strength **must** be developed evenly on both the right and left sides of the body to slow down or eventually stop osteoarthritis deterioration.*

This is how I have lived knee pain-free since 2014.

When you strengthen the body the *right* way, you don't just build muscle; you create a protective shield around every joint you rely on. One thing I want you to notice: when I say, *"Let's strengthen muscles,"*

91

Step Six is all about strengthening **without triggering inflammation**. This is the tricky part, because that's exactly what most strength programs seem to ignore.

If you've undergone a knee replacement, you've probably heard the same refrain: *"Your muscles are weak. You must strengthen them before and after surgery."* Strengthen, strengthen, and… strengthen some more.

The problem is, many people heading into total knee replacement (TKR) are already quite dysfunctional. And by dysfunctional, I mean hip, back, and often shoulder and neck pain can show up like uninvited guests at a party. Yet somehow, the advice is to strengthen muscles in this state of chaos.

This is why, in my programs, strengthening comes *last:* Step Six. By this point, we've tackled inflammation and swelling, ensured your calves, shins, and ankles are moving correctly, addressed flexibility, and eliminated restrictions. We've also implemented the Knee Pain Reduction Strap to help you achieve stability. Essentially, we make sure the right side of your body feels like the left side got the memo and that your stretching and movements are balanced.

I've found that people with knee or hip challenges need to exercise differently. They *cannot* follow the same routines as everyone else, especially if they have osteoarthritis (OA) in the knees or a history of knee injury. Some exercises are downright inappropriate, and ignoring that fact can lead to further knee deterioration.

Now, I'm not here to bash every fitness routine out there. Movement is good. Variety is good. Joy is good.

That said… I do have some thoughts about Zumba.

Zumba is fun. It's energetic. It's great cardio. But knees? Not always thrilled. Why? Zumba involves constant twisting and turning. And remember: knees are hinge joints; they do not swivel like your office chair.

My bigger concern isn't the rhythm; it's the surface. I've seen Zumba classes on piers, grass, sidewalks, parking lots… basically anywhere that makes my knees cringe. Those surfaces might be fine for walking, but frequent pivoting and rotation? Not so much.

Believe it or not, the best surface for Zumba is a basketball court-type floor. Why? Basketball players pivot constantly, and both the court and their shoes are designed to allow it safely. Athletes work with the floor, not against it.

The same principle applies to step classes. Some steps are on rubber mats, and if your shoes have ridges or uneven traction, twisting can create unnecessary stress inside the knee joint. Step classes can be fantastic for strength and conditioning, but only when your surface and footwear are playing on the same team.

I can't tell you how many times I've heard, "I can no longer attend that class because my knees, back, or hips hurt." My hope is that after reading this book, you'll understand why your joints started complaining and make smarter, safer choices in class or life.

Over the past eight years, I've been compiling methods that allow you to strengthen your body, lose weight, and stay active without sacrificing your knees.

You can have fun and build stability while protecting your knees.

Knee Note: Young athletes coming off an injury or looking for prevention will benefit from my ACL manual. Steps one through five of The Moten Method are a must. ACL, MCL, meniscus tears, shin splints, and Osgood-Schlatter disease. These injuries and conditions will benefit from the ACL manual because these individuals are already in shape. They do not have the other joint problems of active adults and seniors.

The key is choosing *how* you move, not whether you move. Routines done on the floor or from a chair can be surprisingly effective.

My osteoarthritis program is one of my most engaging and complete programs. It has everything you need to regain your mobility and strength. (see page 51 for QR code.)

Gym Workouts

When it comes to weight training, dumbbells, barbells, and gym machines are all fair game. The difference is that you won't train like everyone else in the gym, and that's a good thing. Your knees don't need you to prove anything. They need you to move correctly. That may mean slower, more controlled movements and a technique that looks a little different from the person next to you. Think of it as customized care, not limitation.

Safety starts with alignment. In every routine, low-intensity or high-alignment, is your built-in protection system. This is also why instructors benefit from my certification program: learning how to see alignment and cue it properly can prevent years of unnecessary wear and tear. Good coaching doesn't push people harder; it keeps them safer longer.

In the gym, this same principle applies, especially on 45-degree machines. Instead of pushing with both feet at the same time, lower the weight and work one leg at a time. This isn't about making the exercise harder; it's about making it smarter. Alternating legs allows you to identify imbalances and ensures that one side isn't quietly doing all the work while the other side takes a vacation. Once both legs are truly balanced, you can gradually return to using them together.

The same patience applies to machines like the leg curl and leg extension, as well as the inner and outer thigh machines. Work one leg at a time. Give each side your full attention. These machines are valuable tools when used thoughtfully, helping you strengthen each leg correctly and evenly.

Remember, this process isn't about rushing or pushing through pain. It's about protecting your knees, respecting your body, and giving yourself the patience to rebuild stability one smart, aligned movement at a time.

I want to share a story about one of my clients who truly exemplifies this journey. She has been incredible, and through her experience, I've gained a deeper understanding of knee replacements. Many people undergo this surgery, but this particular client required a knee replacement due to four meniscus tears, two on each leg, along with an MCL tear and bone spurs impacting her joint. She was in pain for eight years.

When she first came to me, she was taking six Tylenol pills every day and was understandably miserable and depressed. Despite her condition, she joined my class and was determined. She didn't miss a single session, working out four times a week. Every Friday, we held a big stretching class, and she made sure to attend.

Over time, I observed significant improvements. She could get up and down off the floor, even with her four meniscus tears. At times, she was moving faster than me! She participated in balance coordination, high-intensity aerobics, and chair exercises; she did it all. She continued to work The Moten Method over the next few years.

However, it's important to note that after a while, meniscus tears can start to flip. When they do, they can jam into the joint, making it impossible to bend the knee. This is a critical aspect to understand in managing such injuries.

She was starting to experience a problem. As I mentioned, she had been with me for three and a half years and had been off her drugs during that time.

However, she began to notice that her meniscus tears were affecting her more significantly. She expressed the need for a knee replacement. What happened next was incredible.

Denise had the knee replacement, and the physical therapist advised her to slow down because she was progressing so quickly. She completed steps one, two, and three of her rehabilitation all on her own. The therapist noted that she would finish the program well ahead of others. Essentially, Denise needed to regain the full range of motion in her knee, and she achieved that ahead of schedule.

Within three weeks, Denise returned to class and had nearly full function restored. I was honestly shocked to see her back to full function so soon. She was even able to get back down on the floor after about six weeks and was moving better than before.

I share this story to emphasize a crucial truth: no one should undergo knee replacement surgery without first aligning their body through The Moten Method. It is the most effective program for preparing the body and mind for knee replacement. I've seen it firsthand with Denise and several others who experienced severe bowing of the knees before surgery. Their recovery and results have been nothing short of remarkable.

If you want to avoid the frustration of constantly restarting an exercise program, The Moten Method is where you need to be. It takes time and isn't always easy, but getting better rarely is. One thing I can assure you is that it is absolutely worth your time and effort.

13

SAVING THE NEXT GENERATION OF KNEES

Imagine a twelve-year-old stepping onto a basketball court, lacing up shoes for tryouts, and already wincing. Not from clumsiness. Not from overtraining. But because their knees and hips are already sending warning signs.

I see this far too often. And here's the shocking part: these aren't professional athletes with decades of wear and tear—they're kids. Kids who should be running, jumping, and playing without pain.

I know this firsthand because my daughter trains basketball players ranging from age nine through their early twenties. And as I started evaluating these young athletes, a pattern emerged that made me stop and think: *Why are so many of them already in pain by their teenage years?*

One day, I asked a coach about it. His answer stopped me in my tracks: "When we were kids, we were always outside."

And he was right. We ran around the neighborhood, climbed trees, played kickball, rode bikes, and just… moved. We didn't call it "training"; it was simply life. And those hours of unstructured play built flexible, coordinated, resilient bodies.

I played sports from kindergarten through high school and never suffered a major injury. My daughter followed a similar path and, aside from one ankle sprain, stayed virtually injury-free. The common denominator? We played outside. A lot.

Fast forward to today: kids sit for hours at school, in cars, on couches, and staring at screens, and then we drop them into high-intensity sports and wonder why their knees and hips cry uncle at tryouts. That lack of preparation is not a small issue; it's one of the biggest contributors to the injuries I see.

Parents, this is your wake-up call. The right foundation now can help your child stay safe, competitive, and most importantly, pain-free.

To understand why this matters so much, we need to look at what's happening inside a young athlete's body. In particular, I want to talk about boys between the ages of thirteen and twenty, what I call the "painful years." During this phase, growth spurts happen fast. Bones lengthen rapidly, while muscles and tendons struggle to keep up. The result? Tightness, poor alignment, and joints, especially knees and hips, are taking the hit.

And that's where the real trouble begins.

As a result, the tendons, which attach to the bones, are not keeping pace. This discrepancy creates friction and tension around the joints, particularly in the knees, which can lead to pain even before the child starts participating in any sports.

The challenge I want to discuss is called Osgood-Schlatter syndrome. Although some refer to it as a disease, I prefer the term "syndrome." Osgood-Schlatter syndrome occurs when a child experiences rapid growth, especially in the shin bone (the tibia);

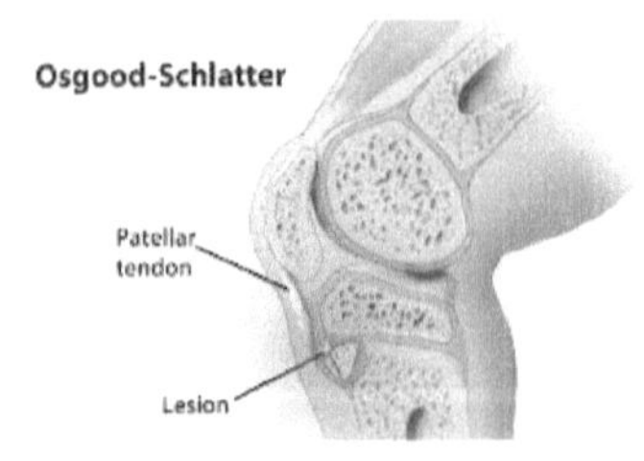

while the child's bones are getting longer, the patellar tendon does not stretch as fast, creating this tug-of-war with the bony bump of the tibial tubercle. This discrepancy causes the patellar tendon to pull on the knee, leading to pain.

Knee Note: *Osgood-Schlatter syndrome can be easily avoided if children adopt stretching routines early in their teens.*

Boys, in particular, may face additional challenges because their tendons and ligaments tend to have less elasticity, making them less flexible. During growth spurts, boys can experience knee problems due to this lack of flexibility, alongside the rapid growth of bones. As boys develop, increases in testosterone can also lead to decreased flexibility in their tendons and ligaments. This often results in strains and injuries during early adolescence.

It's crucial for parents of boys aged thirteen to twenty who are getting involved in sports to prioritize flexibility training. Enrolling them in local studios or programs that focus on flexibility can help prepare their bodies for the demands of competitive sports. If young athletes are involved with intense athletic activities without proper preparation, they risk injuries that could lead to long-term issues, including arthritis or osteoarthritis.

From ages sixteen to eighteen, some young athletes are introduced to anti-inflammatory medications like Advil, which I find not in the best interest of the child. These kids are not professional athletes, so if they miss a game, they will not lose any pay. While they may attract attention from college scouts, it is counterproductive to rely on medication for pain management at such a young age. Long-term use of Advil can lead to serious health issues, such as stomach ulcers.

At this stage, young male athletes experience increased tenderness and stiffness in their tendons and ligaments, which further contribute to reduced flexibility. Additionally, growth plates, the soft tissue between bones that enable growth, are present at this age. If a child is injured while playing contact sports like football and their growth plates are damaged, it can lead to complications later in life.

Though injuries to growth plates are not always catastrophic, they are certainly avoidable. It's important to consider the risks of young children playing high-impact sports before their bodies are adequately prepared.

We want to prevent these kids from living in pain. I've seen many cases, especially among basketball players who suffer from ACL and PCL tears. These injuries can affect them for the rest of their lives. We need to make better choices to prepare these kids before they attend tryouts for any sports, particularly high-intensity ones.

It's crucial to get them moving beforehand. Additionally, during the off-season, they should engage in different sports that do not repeatedly overuse the same muscles.

For example, if a child is involved in basketball, why not introduce them to swimming, Pilates, or some type of exercise class? Swimming can relieve joint tension, and weight training can help as well, provided it diversifies their muscle use. Activities like dance can also be beneficial. It might sound unconventional, but it's essential for kids to engage different muscles, especially when participating in basketball or soccer.

To ensure your child transitions into adulthood without chronic pain, it's important to rotate them through various sports at different times to protect their joints. This is the fundamental principle.

Girls

Now, let's discuss girls. Their development is slightly different from that of boys. Girls between the ages of thirteen and twenty experience significant hormonal shifts with the onset of their menstrual cycles.

Girls tend to experience growth spurts earlier than boys, typically between ages eleven and fourteen, after which they generally stop growing, while boys may have longer and later growth spurts. Additionally, the estrogen girls produce can make their ligaments more flexible, which does set them up for injuries in the future.

Training Philosophy: A Paradigm Shift for Female Athletes

The way we train young female athletes must evolve. For too long, traditional sports conditioning has followed a male-centered model that overlooks the unique biomechanics, hormonal influences, and movement patterns of girls. My training philosophy is built on creating a paradigm shift, one that prioritizes alignment, kinetic chain, flexibility, stability, and movement control before power, speed, and endurance.

Basketball players could benefit from Zumba classes to use their hips and create flexibility in the ankles. Ballet can enhance grace, posture, and controlled transitions, skills that improve stability, balance, and spatial awareness.

Female athletes deserve training that works *with* their bodies, not against them. That means emphasizing balance, posture, and proper landing mechanics, the same foundational skills taught in gymnastics, to develop body awareness and protect the knees from unnecessary strain. The focus is not on how much weight they can lift or how fast they can run, but on how efficiently they move through space and absorb impact.

This approach could restore what's been missing in female sports training: the connection between gymnastics, ballet, Zumba, and the kinetic chain.

It's important to understand that ligaments in women and girls tend to be a bit looser, especially during their menstrual cycle. This looser structure is a significant reason why they do experience more injuries than boys. So, what can be done about this?

Knee Note: Ligaments attach a bone to a bone. The knee is one of the largest joints in the body, with four ligaments that do not stretch.

First, it's essential to introduce girls to sports early on and focus on flexibility. While girls are generally more flexible than boys, it's also crucial to strengthen the ankles, shins, calves, and feet to create a solid foundation for the sports they play.

During childhood, physical activity improves children's body awareness, control, and balance. According to the Mayo Clinic, strength training can be incorporated into a fitness plan as early as age seven or eight.[1]

Additionally, girls often face challenges with muscle tone. They tend to gain muscle more slowly than boys, underscoring the need for early and consistent stability and strengthening exercises. Testosterone, which helps boys develop muscle faster, is less prevalent in girls due to higher estrogen levels. One physical indicator of higher estrogen is typically wider hips. While this characteristic is natural, it can lead to misalignments in the knees, increasing the likelihood of injuries.

Before enrolling your child in sports, it's vital to consider how to keep them safe. Popular activities like volleyball, basketball, and soccer involve extensive jumping, twisting, and turning, which can increase injury risks for girls.

> ***Knee Note:*** *Preparing girls for their sports using boxing classes, playing ping pong while switching hands, and Zumba and Pilates taught by good instructors.*

Water workouts are highly effective and can help girls and boys build strength without placing undue stress on their bodies. Practices such as running, aerobic classes, or other activities in the water are not only enjoyable but also easier on their joints compared to traditional gym workouts.

Prioritizing proper preparation and strength training can greatly reduce the risk of these injuries and promote a healthier, more active lifestyle for young athletes.

---

[1]. Mayo Clinic Staff, "Strength Training: OK for Kids?," Mayo Clinic, December 15, 2023, https://www.mayoclinic.org/healthy-lifestyle/tween-and-teen-health/in-depth/strength-training/art-20047758.

It's important to understand that certain injuries can occur in children if they aren't careful, often due to a lack of stretching. The first step to preventing these issues is to ensure they stretch regularly.

Stretching is essential, not optional, especially for conditions like Sever's disease, which commonly affects kids who enjoy jumping and can lead to heel pain.

I've worked with clients like Rachel, a ballet dancer who developed bunions from being in ballet classes at a young age. When you have bunions, it can alter your gait. Rachel began to walk incorrectly, and over time, she experienced hip pain that persisted for about five or six years. Since her walking pattern was affected, this also led to knee pain.

I met her after her knee pain was disrupting her cycling.

After a month of trying to alleviate her pain without success, I realized there might be an underlying issue. Her mother recommended an MRI, not just for her knee but also for her hip. The MRI revealed that she had torn the labrum in her hip, which was contributing to her knee problems. After her hip was repaired, her knee pain went away.

This situation illustrates how an initial hip injury in a ballet dancing class escalated into a knee problem.

Our children depend on us not just to cheer from the sidelines but to guide them toward a future where their bodies are strong, resilient, and pain-free. Most parents do what they believe is right: they rely on medical advice to determine when their child should play, rest, or return after an injury. That trust is understandable. But it is no longer enough.

The truth is, we are asking young bodies to perform at elite levels without first giving them a solid physical foundation. And when pain shows up, the solution addresses the symptom, not the system.

The Moten Method was created to change that. It was designed to build a lifelong movement foundation for both children and adults, one that respects joint health, restores balance, and protects the knees and hips before pain becomes a permanent companion. This is not about pushing harder. It's about moving smarter, earlier, and with intention.

I know this system works because I lived the alternative. I injured my ankle at thirty-three, and the treatment I received in 1990 is essentially the same advice being offered to young athletes in 2026. Same protocols. Same instructions. Same outcomes. Decades later, we are still reacting to pain instead of preventing it.

Our kids deserve better than recycled solutions for modern problems. They deserve guidance that honors how their bodies grow, move, and adapt. If we change the way we prepare them today, we can protect their knees, preserve their confidence, and give them a future where movement is a source of joy.

14
FINAL REFLECTIONS
WHY KNEES?

Of all the things to become captivated by, really, knees? I understand being obsessed with something glamorous, like shoes, but the knee has always captured my attention like nothing else.

In 1992, I refused painkillers for my right knee. That simple choice ignited a curiosity that has never stopped burning inside me.

Perhaps it's because I witnessed my sister and mother lose their health and mobility due to medication.

What drives me to search for the ultimate remedy for knee pain around the world is straightforward: I want to stop osteoarthritis in its tracks. Yes, I said it. My goal is to halt the slow, silent deterioration that robs people of mobility, joy, and freedom.

For years, I repeated a mantra: there has to be another way. I remember early in my career stating that I didn't want to rely on any drugs because if I did find a solution, I wouldn't recognize it if I were under the influence of medication. I never took any drugs or shots, and I definitely never underwent surgery, because I believed there had to be another way.

That stubborn belief and unwavering faith are what led me to write this book. The similarities of so many people struggling with knee pain became impossible to ignore. After hearing their stories, I could almost predict what they were feeling. It was as if they were unknowingly part of a silent "I Got Knee Pain Too" movement of knee pain, a movement no one asked to join.

I became determined to find a remedy for my knee pain, which morphed into a movement against an industry that doesn't focus on healing. I wrote this book because I want everyone to know that I hear you, I see you, and I understand your pain.

You are not alone. You are part of the "I Got Knee Pain Too" movement, so I hope you've seen reflections of your own journey in these chapters, not just to relieve your pain but to finally understand it.

Why do we endure pain for one year, five years, or even ten years? Here's the truth I have learned over two decades of hurting, healing, and refusing to give up: pain does not have the final say. You do.

In 2014, my knees became pain-free. Since that day, I have shared my experiences and insights with men and women around the world. For you, this is only the beginning.

This book is dedicated to anyone who refuses to live in pain. My hope is that it empowers you to choose real healing over mere pain management. You deserve better, and so do your knees.

I created a quote about twenty years ago that sums it up: "When you take care of your knees, your knees will carry you for a lifetime."

THANK YOU FOR READING MY BOOK!

Note from the Knee Keeper:
Just to say thanks for buying and reading my book,

Scan the QR Code to get my eBook:
"Unlocking the Secrets to Knee Pain"
and use code MYKNEE:

I appreciate your interest in my book and value your feedback, as it helps me improve future versions. I would appreciate it if you could leave your invaluable review on Amazon.com with your feedback.
Thank you!